HEAL

*a year's worth of improvements
to run an excellent healthcare organization*

By A P Palmer

Copyright © 2011 A P Palmer

All rights reserved.
This book, or parts thereof,
may not be reproduced in any form without permission

ISBN 978-1463663575

HEAL

*a year's worth of improvements
to run an excellent healthcare organization*

For Hannah & Sam

Introduction

Why can't we have healthcare excellence? What's holding back healthcare organizations from creating facilities, services, and environments that have the look and feel of a Four Seasons, the seamless operations of Disneyland, the ambiance of Starbuck's *third place*, or the innovations of IDEO?

Yes, healthcare is more complex; indeed, it has more moving parts, players, and egos. All the more reason, then, for Zen simplicity and quality, of quiet leadership and confidence. Excellence for those critical, and always emotional, moments in our lives, with the personal, attentive care that nurtures and heals, in place of the high stress, chaos, and low touch that can frighten, intimidate, and weaken even the strongest souls.

HEAL presents a year of hard-won insights and challenges experienced in the healthcare world, each dedicated to identifying and overcoming the individual and institutional barriers to a first-rate and exceptional healthcare environment—an environment that nurtures, supports, and delivers care and compassion for its patients, colleagues, and communities.

Use it well.

1
Customer Care

WELCOME.

Every hotel and restaurant worth its Zagat rating has a doorperson, a highly visible concierge whose single responsibility is to welcome each and every guest who arrives at the main entrance, at every hour of its operating day. A simple yet powerful task it is - to offer a friendly, personal greeting and always, to meet one of the most basic human needs: acknowledgement. With that acknowledgement, the concierge starts the invisible task of hand-offs so critical in healthcare organizations, setting in motion the quality personal interactions your guests want and need to experience for a satisfying visit.

So, does your organization have a concierge? Hire one, more than one, and position them at your main entrance, to own the task of acknowledging your guests, patients, partners, and helping them get to where they need to be, even if it's simply directions to the reception area

Make it SIMPLE to get here from there.

Does your hospital still use the colored lines on the linoleum hallway floors to direct patients and guests from the reception area to imaging, the lab or to administration? Yellow to imaging, red to the emergency department, dotted black to administration. It's like following a subway map - without a subway!

Instead of relying on or reinventing the visuals of a past modern era, use words, simple graphics and your readily available resource, humans. Clear signage is critical, as are concierge and escort services (in addition to it being every employee's job, right?), and valets. A few important but simple, non-competing signs. Staffed reception areas at public entrances. Uncomplicated patient registration. Excellent phone and messaging services. An easy to use, uncluttered website, with meaningful online tools.

There are plenty of opportunities to help your guests get there from here, to where they need to be when they visit your facilities and services, in person or virtually. Make getting there clear and simple.

Create
MOMENTS of Truth.

What is excellence? Quality, distinction, commitment and compassion.

What is the opposite of excellence? Anything else: mediocrity. How do you know excellence? Is it a vague Supreme Court definition: you'll know it when you see it? Is it based on what you can measure, your core measures, HCAHPS or Press Ganey scores?

Isn't excellence those little, unheralded events that happen to you, your guests, your staff in the course of the day: the warm greeting at the front door;

the clinician waiting a solid 18-seconds before speaking; sitting with a family member in a private setting instead of in a crowded waiting room; always acknowledging staff anxiety and grief?

These are your organization's Moments of Truth.

Excellence is paying attention to the Moments of Truth that are everywhere in your organization, preparing for them to pop up. It's giving them the air and opportunity to happen, so excellence becomes the norm, and not the exception.

Be a guest with a physical CHALLENGE for a day.

Grab a wheelchair from the concierge or valet and check out your facility for the day. Navigate through the hospital or clinic in your new vehicle, from the reception desk, to registration, on to the outpatient clinics, the ED, maybe even up to the floors. What's it like? Are the hallways and ramps clear, uncluttered, wide enough, easy to navigate solo, uncluttered? Do the elevators and lifts work for you without assistance?

Try getting around your cafeteria: don't ask for help, but notice if anyone, especially your staff, offers to assist if you need it.

How about getting into and out of the public restrooms . . . can you do it on your own? Do the automatic door openers work? Are the sinks and towel dispensers easy to reach?

Anything that frustrates you or doesn't get you where you need to be during this excursion is broken. Don't assume it will get easier with practice. Imagine its impact on your guests who need to rely on them for their daily navigation.

If anything's frustrating to you, it's broken. Fix it now.

LOYALTY comes with quality care.

Ask yourself this question: why do you return over and over to some businesses and services, but not to others? What is it about the places you are loyal to that keep you coming back, that come immediately to mind when friends and family ask for the best XYZ services? Is it the intangible qualities of its reputation, its look and feel, or the tangible quality of its products and services, the consistent ratings and facts? Is it the quality of the people who deliver the service?

It's doubtless a combination of all of the above; but it all boils down to consistently high quality. Reliable, focused, superior excellence that is delivered to everyone, and at every conceivable entry point, from its marketing, real and virtual, phone and front door greeting to the follow-up, website resources, and next visits.

Excellent quality is how you generate loyalty. It's easy. And it's difficult. But it's well worth it.

Cell-phone ETIQUETTE equals integrity.

Cell phones. They've become a human appendage: we reach for them, unconsciously, with little effort to restrain either their presence or our response. There's a story of a surgeon upbraiding his staff for calling his cell while he was in surgery; so many chances to avoid the situation (turn it off? leave it in his locker?), but its active presence was nothing more than a piece of his uniform, his person, no more or less important than his scrubs.

Cell phones are a love/hate relationship in business and life. Just don't let them get in the way of providing exceptional patient and guest care.

In patient care, the presence of cell phones, particularly those with cameras, can create an unsafe and unethical environment. They open up opportunities to interrupt care, as one impulsively reaches for a vibrating phone while attending to a patient or dispensing medication. Cell phones present thoughtless ways to violate privacy and undermine the unique relationship with patients and coworkers.

HIPAA is the least of your worries. Your patient's care is at stake, and so is your integrity.

Create a patient and visitor LIBRARY.

Welcome and enable your patients and guests as partners in their own healthcare by creating a library and learning center, both in your facility (remember, not everyone has computer access), as well as through your website or online presence.

Set aside a convenient and highly visible space in your facility. Equip it with the latest and best tools and resources to engage and satisfy curiosity and the need to learn about health and wellness. Make it especially friendly to non-clinical visitors, with extreme consideration to their health literacy needs. But never patronize. Provide age-specific materials, especially those that address adult-learning methodologies and needs. Above all, make it interesting, fun, and easy to access.

Web access, medical journal subscriptions, and basic alternative learning tools are the minimum requirements. Interactive and multi-media applications, introduction to cloud-based resources, and high-quality educational partnerships are valuable key components.

Turn it into a *third-place*, near the cafeteria, and guests and staff can mingle and learn. Cool.

Healthcare is a FOREIGN language.

Every industry has its own language and terminology, unique to insiders, but not interchangeable with other industries, and rarely shared with the public.

Healthcare's foreignness might top them all; it touches so many of us. Your everyday clinical terminology is normal at work, between clinicians and staff, but it can be a struggle for your guests (probably some of your staff, too, but they may be reluctant to admit to it).

Health literacy is a major safety and quality issue. Patients are asked to be more involved with their own care but they are at an enormous disadvantage: they may lack an educational or working background to be anything more than a "patient." Clinical terminology, acronyms, the quick shorthand language of healthcare workers are a mystery - it's a language virtually unknown outside your walls, except on as-seen-on-TV medical dramas, Pharma ads, and on too many to count websites. It's still foreign.

Take the time to simplify and translate your message to your patients with common, every day terms and language. It's a good way to improve communication, patient care and, a big plus here, to increase compliance.

The payoff? Everyone will think you're great.

Teach SERVICE recovery.

Healthcare is the people business. And with people, there will always be a chance to do service recovery, to fix an error, improve communication, or to undo harm.

When a clinician is running late, it's vital to keep everyone, especially the next patients, updated and reassured often. When insurance won't cover an expensive procedure, prepare to offer an alternative that either is covered or will be less money out of pocket.

Be prepared for the inevitable and anticipate the unexpected by empowering your staff with simple scripts and responses. They can deliver a service recovery response as a confident offer to help instead of opening up a defensive run to the lawyer.

Everyone should work in FOOD SERVICE at least once in their life.

If you work with people (almost everyone does), food service is the best training ground to learn some of life's most valuable skills.

Attention everyone: get off the pedestal.

At its best and its worst, waiting tables, serving customers, and working a commercial or industrial kitchen will teach a well-rounded curriculum of humility, assertiveness, respect, ego, the value of holistic teamwork, and, above all, the power of the weak: the next time you think about being rude to a waiter, especially before your food arrives, remember: Revenge will be his.

Embrace the CRITIC.

You will always learn from the critic, the naysayer, definitely more than you will from your supporters.

Everyone loves glowing comments and praise. Too much of a good thing, though, can lead to complacency and it's hard to make improvements when you are resting on your laurels.

When someone offers criticism or suggestions, get more information from them. Consider the source; some people love to complain, just for the fun of it. But many others may have an important issue you can recognize as an opportunity for you to improve.

Don't wallow in the negative or let the group become defensive. Seek out the ways to use what you hear and then make things better.

FOLLOW-UP on every patient visit.

Never let a single patient visit go without a follow-up call. Ever.

Designate a few people within every service to call each patient within 24 hours of their visit, regardless of the type of visit. It goes without saying that it is a chance to improve customer satisfaction. A follow-up call is also an excellent chance to encourage compliance, to answer forgotten or embarrassing questions, to hear about unmet needs or unexpected complications, and to make follow-up appointments or referrals.

Follow-up calls are a basic opportunity to provide better care, communication, and always, to extend kindness and compassion.

Always say, "PLEASE" and "THANK YOU."

Kindergarten rules apply to adults, too, not just 5-year-olds—probably more so (where do they learn it, anyway?) There are a lot of reasons and opportunities to say "please" and "thank you" to your patients, coworkers, leaders, staff, and guests.

Barking orders or demanding action are not guaranteed to gain compliance, to win many friends, or to influence most people. Saying "please" is not a sign of begging. It smoothes the way, opens up communication, instills trust and cooperation. Followed by a "thank you," you've got a perfect recipe for a more comfortable transaction.

Add a "thank you" note or comment to billing statements, to community and in-house marketing materials, even on the patient's food tray—a simple, hand-written note is a touch of the human hand in a chaotic environment.

The patient EXPERIENCE is everyone's job.

Promote a system-wide investment in making the patient experience your #1 goal. Put it in the water.

Physicians, nurses, lab techs, environmental services, food service, administrators, vendors and consultants: make sure everyone owns the responsibility to create an excellent experience for every patient and their guests.

24 / 7 / 365

Healthcare is a round the clock enterprise, even with sleeping patients and a skeleton crew. Everyone on your staff has to be engaged the minute they step into their role whether it's at 7am, 7pm, or 2am.

It's show time, all the time, in healthcare. If you can't show up, then get off the stage, find support, and let the understudy take over.

Staff: You've got to be present, be there whatever the shift.

Leaders: You've got to support them - completely and consistently, and let them know it.

A man without a smiling face must not open a shop. (Chinese Proverb)

Patients, families, and guests are not BARRIERS to overcome.

Just like children at a school and customers in a restaurant, your patients and guests are the only reason for your organization to exist.

Patients and guests are not a barrier or nuisance, something in the way of your staff getting its work done. They are your work.

Never forget it.

It's okay to say, "I'm SORRY."

Being able to say, "I'm sorry," can have a big impact on your relationships, even in the healthcare environment.

"I'm sorry" doesn't have to mean you are responsible or guilty of doing something wrong; when you say it sincerely, with consideration and thoughtfulness, it honestly means you regret that something unfortunate has happened to someone you care about.

"I'm sorry" can clear the way to a deeper, more open discussion about what happened and where to go from here. It may also lessen the antagonism that can crop up when the unexpected, or the unfortunate, does happen. It may reduce unnecessary visits to a lawyer.

Focus on HUMAN-centered practices.

Patient care gowns and blankets, building and landscape design, curb appeal and building aesthetics, clinical services, community and professional outreach, ergonomic working environments; pay attention to the basic needs of the humans you care for who are receiving and giving care.

Please: don't pay more attention to the needs of the new EHR or da Vinci tools than you do to your people. Easy to do, but it's not worth the effort in the overall health of your organization.

Pay attention to the humans.

How do you get INTO your facility?

Patient and guest access should be easy, seamless, smooth and simple. The front door, the website, the phone. Clear and seamless.

Imagine you are Disneyland, where the operational hard work is done behind and below the scenes, and everyone is in charge of making the customer experience the best possible experience they've had.

Whether it's patient referrals from community clinics or inpatient admits from the emergency department, make patient and guest access effortless, uncomplicated, with the effort and inner workings virtually invisible to your patients and guests.

2
Emotions

PERCEPTION is reality.

The image of your organization can say more than the reality of your organization. Do your guests, whether they are your patients, staff, vendors or the neighbors, feel welcomed and cared for when they visit? Are they confident that you care about the quality of the services you provide, that you deliver the highest quality of care, and that you guarantee their safety and the best possible outcomes?

Your guests' reality starts with the look and feel of the buildings and the grounds, the acknowledgement paid to them when they arrive at the front door or the emergency department or outpatient clinics. Their reality starts from the word on the street, or the comments from your partners and competitors to your patients and customers in the community.

Show your guests, staff, and customers and community that you care. You might not get a second chance to tell them.

Reward and RECOGNITION aren't just for sales people.

We are all like sales people - we love to be recognized for the work we do, for showing up, and trying hard to succeed. For the successes and the gallant attempts.

Take plenty of opportunities to recognize and celebrate the little moments of your staff's achievements, as individuals and as teams. The events above and beyond, the milestones in individual lives, the hard falls from a valiant effort.

Make rewards and recognition practices meaningful and authentic; spread it wide, even with your physicians, managers and leaders.

The patient experience is always EMOTIONAL.

You may want your patients to be as rational, logical and attentive as you, your services, your clinicians, and plans.

It's simply not possible. Patients arrive anxious, focused on their (your) environment, and will respond to everything that happens to them based on their emotions. Their decisions will be based on their emotional needs and perceptions.

So, acknowledge this reality. Be prepared to meet their emotional needs with warmth, comfort, and softness. With patience, more communication, quiet moments, and reassurance.

Reduce the COMPLEXITY.

Healthcare is big, strange, intense, noisy, clinical, detached. It's complex. There are unrelenting noises from machines and procedures; the hard, cold feel of instruments that are touched and touch back; ambient odors, offensive and chemical; the unfiltered, too bright, and unnatural light; the alien language and terminology of healthcare; the stale air; and hordes of unknown people doing unthinkable tasks.

Make the care personal. Graceful. Open. Human.

Communicate. Reduce the effort needed to make it all work; move it in the opposite direction.

Any intelligent fool can make things bigger and more complex...
It takes a touch of genius - and a lot of courage to move in the opposite direction.
Albert Einstein

Expect RESISTANCE to change.

Status quo is comfortable, predictable, and safe. Change is scary, unknown, and uncomfortable. Expect resistance with every change, every new color, and every new idea, every new seating arrangement.

Expect some to take it personally, needing space to adjust, to fit it into their worldview.

Expect resistance. Don't let it surprise you. Simply clear the path for everyone to be able to do their work.

Provide clear and consistent communication, encouragement, and the opportunity to make the change their own.

QUALITY is emotional.

There are ever-increasing metrics around healthcare and its quality, but it's important to understand that quality is also a feeling, an emotion. Quality is a place that feels clean and fresh, where the lights are on, music or noise is subtle, communication is open and civil, care is appropriate and timely, and rumors are minimal. It feels personal and comfortable.

Quality is calm and confident.

Quality is emotional, irrational, but it is real.

Quality is a safe, well-organized and excellent environment. It's like a spa, a well-appointed and elegant hotel. It's the comfort of one's personal space.

Comfort, care and quality are assured.

Trying to change a culture is a FOOL'S errand.

It's never a good idea to patronize an organization's culture. It's guaranteed to set up defensiveness and resistance, especially if you are a new leader, visiting clinician, or consultant.

When something isn't working in a way you are familiar with or expect, it's easy to want to change the culture. Instead, focus on behavior change, not culture change.

If an organization needs to improve patient care outcomes, its care delivery standards, or relationship performance, start with a focus on changing the specific behaviors and actions that are demonstrated to lead to poor outcomes.

Don't focus on changing the culture.

Work from the ground up, the grassroots, to identify actions that may be creating unacceptable performance or care, and then concentrate on specific behaviors to replace them. Build on excellent behaviors to create new strengths.

It's always PERSONAL.

Healthcare: it's always personal.

A woman's mammogram doesn't get much more personal. Nor does open-heart surgery.

A patient's reaction to a lab report or a clinician's to her board results: it's always personal.

Create an environment that allows for, that demands, a space for the personal. Build an environment that is thoughtful and considerate of the personal needs that are everywhere in your organization, the facility and the environment.

Make personal what you stand for, who you are.

Here. NOW.

Like Moments of Truth, Here is the most important place to be. Now.

Here is mindfulness, being present right now, instead of being elsewhere, anywhere but here. This patient; this meeting. Now.

Here is paying attention to the people you are with, your role and your responsibility to that interaction. This surgery; this pathology report. Now.

Here is paying attention to the look, feel, smell, light, temperature, essence, emotions of the here and now.

A lot goes into the here and now, but it all comes together when you commit to it.

Cultivate an organization of mutual TRUST.

How disheartening to attend an operational meeting of managers and directors, chaperoned by an equal number of their CxOs —who expressly state they don't trust that their staff can come up with appropriate plans for the work required.

Lesson to leaders: If you don't trust your staff to do their work, you have a huge problem, one that involves more than simply replacing them or micromanaging. Your creating learned helplessness, and more.

Micromanaging will never solve the problems you want solved.

Micromanaging is the perfect way to erode trust, and to build a culture of learned helplessness. If your staff doesn't leave your organization out of frustration, they will learn to sit back and wait for you to do their work for them. What a waste.

Is DRAMA the norm?

Hospitals can be funny places in a crisis: many operate more smoothly and without drama during a crisis, accomplishing everything that needs to be done without error.

Why? When professionalism kicks in, processes are followed, checklists are monitored, muscle memory takes over, egos are pulled in, and the drama of personal back-stories has no room when immediate patient care is the focus.

You don't want a crisis everyday. But this knowledge can be a creative challenge to build improvements into your clinical processes as well as into your interpersonal and Emotional Quotient skill set.

Learn to identify the drama centers and create an atmosphere to move beyond it.

What you do
is about LIFE.

Everything that happens in healthcare organizations, to patients, their families and visitors, to staff and the guests who walk through the doors, has to do with their life, their emotions.

Whether it's the personal service, the human touch, or the highest technical procedure, people are ultimately less interested in how equipment works than in how it made them feel; how it will affect their life.

Healthcare is all about life. Make it what you are about.

Show RESPECT to those who will be most affected by a new initiative.

When you add new processes or tools, like technology or equipment, learn to understand and appreciate how it will impact those most immediately involved, whether it will be the physicians and clinicians or the frontline staff. Many tech changes don't make life any simpler or easier for anyone, either in the short or long term.

Remember to always include the end-user as a critical partner in your planning and rollout processes. You don't want to spend valuable time with end-users who passively resist when you could have engaged their assistance in the beginning. You don't want to waste time, after the fact, mending fences or jerry-rigging to make a new process or product work the way it was designed to.

BULLYING doesn't happen only on the playground.

Does bullying have to be part of the nature of the healthcare beast? Enabled by tradition, work silos, and the healthcare power and financial hierarchy, it seems inevitable.

But it doesn't have to be. It can be reduced if not eliminated.

First, and most importantly, call bullying by its real name. That's a vital good first start.

Second, leadership is key, both at the clinical and non-clinical levels. Hold everyone accountable for her and his behavior and interactions. Stop bullying in its tracks.

Third, a safe environment to open up communication and allow assertiveness to become valued is essential. Staff relationship and communication skill development are invaluable in healthcare settings. Make safety and communication a priority, and make sure it's available house-wide.

Give positive
REINFORCEMENT
for excellence.
Early and often.

Reinforce and encourage the performance you expect from your staff and partners. Pay attention to the behaviors and outcomes that serve them and your healthcare environment well.

Acknowledge simple actions, the helping hand and compassion, as well as the one-offs: going the extra mile for a frightened or lonely patient with a Skype connection to far-away family. Celebrating a hard-won night shift with your department's perpetual nemesis with a midnight barbecue.

Everyone is responsible for a group's excellent performance. And every excellent performance is a cause for encouragement and a lot of reinforcement.

Stop YELLING.

In the course of a typical day in intense and emotional environments like healthcare, miscommunication can easily lapse into chaos, tempers, loud voices, accusations and blame. Whether it's on the floors, in the nursing station or hallways, the cafeteria or private offices, patients, guests, and staff will hear and sense it all. You are not alone here; it's not your space alone.

Loud voices, yelling, and chaos are stressful, disrespectful, and unnerving to everyone around, and the upshot is an unhealthy and unsafe environment at best; a dangerous one at its worst.

Though it feels like it, this isn't middle school anymore, friends. Be civil, be professional, be grownups. Save the drama for your own time.

Care for your CAREGIVERS.

One of the toughest jobs in the world is taking care of people who are ill, who are hurt or vulnerable, or who are dying. Care-giving can be rewarding, but it is definitely a stressful, frequently thankless, and often unhealthy job.

The best, most compassionate members of your staff need respite, recognition and an occasional change of scenery and duties.

Take good care of your staff, volunteers and partners, those who take care. Celebrate their accomplishments and good works; acknowledge their personal anxiety and grief. Pay attention to signs of compassion fatigue, signs that they may be burning out, are overloaded with the sickest of the sick, the anxiety of the worried well or, that they may possibly be in the wrong business.

Nurture your staff as they care for your business, your patients and themselves. Give them respite, room to breathe, to refresh and regroup.

Respect the POWER of gossip and rumor.

Gossip and rumors run rampant in healthcare. And it often reflects the psychological health of your organization.

If you want to get a sense and the temperature of your place, stay tuned-in to the latest round and sources of gossip, from who's who on the grapevine, to the water-cooler topic of the day.

Keeping your ears tuned in to gossip and rumor is a great way to gauge business dynamics, to anticipate brilliant opportunities or problems, to uncover or preempt crises, to discover the new leaders and alpha members of the staff, and to adjust feedback and responses if necessary.

And whether it's fear of regulators, mergers, or layoffs, or the latest news of a coworker's professional crisis, fear can be contagious. Keep a finger on the pulse to limit its impact.

Be the sponge. Don't become part of the problem and pass along anything you hear. Be the one to stop a fire from spreading.

3 Leadership

LISTEN up.

Listening is a core competency of leaders in high-quality organizations, and no less so than in healthcare.

Listen to your staff, your coworkers, customers, partners and patients, your staff and community. Never assume you know what they think or mean without being available to listen to them, to really hear their stories.

When they speak, listen more than you talk. Remember, it's about them; it's not about you.

Don't forget the 18-second rule: after you meet, learn to be quiet, to not talk, for at least 18 seconds. Resist the urge to jump in to fill the uncomfortable silence. You will be surprised what you find out.

Be still and listen.

… Take your staff
to LUNCH.

Or to coffee, or breakfast, or drinks after work. Whatever the schedule allows. But always make sure your schedule will allow it.

You will be amazed what you can learn when you regularly treat members of your staff to one-on-one time, offsite and casual.

Whether it's new insight into what makes her tick, learning the latest run of the mill water-cooler gossip, or hearing new and innovative ideas for business improvement, casual breaks outside of the routine are a perfect way to connect with the people you supervise.

And, being the good leader you hope to be, it's a great way to coach and mentor, to support and build the best team.

Set a good EXAMPLE.

Just as children pick up their parent's good habits and bad, your staff will undoubtedly pick up and mirror your own values and leadership style.

It's just as important as it sounds. Your mom was right (she's always right): Do your best, be nice, respect your coworkers, be on time, pay attention, listen to your peers and colleagues and staff, teach what you know, and take initiative.

Leaders are role models. They set the tone. Good and bad.

PhD Leadership - short course:
Make a list of all the things that you abhor; don't do them to others - ever.
Make a list of all the things done to you that you love; do them to others - always.
Dee Hock (VISA)

Stop listening to the sound of your own VOICE.

Executives, managers and team leaders: stop monopolizing meetings or conversations with your staff and constituents. Give others a chance to make a point or suggest an idea. Offer the floor, ask questions, solicit opinions and ask for feedback.

You'll always learn twice as much about your organization if you listen to your staff, guests and patients. They have much to offer. That's why you hired them in the first place.

MANAGE down as well as up.

'Managing up' is a popular business school mantra that is meant to instill the value of taking initiative and to help make the boss more successful. It's personal drive; the tasks you do above and beyond.

'Managing down,' on the other hand, is less often talked about but is equally if not more valuable. A managers' job is to lead, to communicate, mentor, communicate, influence, teach, communicate, empower, recognize, communicate, value, trust, promote and sponsor. Share what you know from meetings, seminars. Teach what you know from more experience, from more knowledge and more insight.

Don't be bossy and don't expect your staff to be at your beck and call. Let them do their work. Just do your job exceptionally well so those you supervise can learn from you how to do theirs.

TRUST.

It goes without saying: It is vital that leadership be both trusting and trustworthy.

Be fair, clear and consistent. Trust your people to do their job knowing your expectations, goals, and values.

Be a role model. Model exceptional behavior, standards, ethics, and work/life balance.

Be open and available. As a leader, you have wisdom and experience to pass along. So pass it along.

Allow for honest and remediable mistakes without retribution. Let your people do their jobs without fear of failure.

Don't play favorites and never, ever, be cliquish. Mingle. Be fair.

RESPECT your staff and show it.

Respect their time, talent, commitment to their work and to the organization. Pay them well; provide opportunities for career and professional growth; reward initiative. Don't patronize.

Always respect their work environment. Give them an atmosphere that complements the demands and requirements of their work. Provide the best, most appropriate tools to perform their work both ergonomically and effectively.

Respect their need for recognition. A job well done is never to go unnoticed. Ditto birthdays, anniversaries, personal milestones and events.

If you don't, or can't, treat your staff with trust and respect, you're a fool to be surprised when they suffer poor morale or leave for greener pastures. Quid pro quo.

Manage by WALKING around.

This has long been one of the best pieces of management advice out there. Wouldn't you know it: it has a natural home in the healthcare industry.

It's also called rounding.

Set up a no-exceptions hour commitment each and every day, say from 7-8am, or 11-noon. Then, just wander the halls; check out the cafeteria, the coffee regulars; scrub up and observe the early surgery suite; visit the newborn nursery. Get to know your staff. Reacquaint yourself with new and established leaders. Spend some time with patients and guests.

Let everybody see your friendly face!

In fact, every leadership coach you talk with should emphasize walking around, rounding, huddling, or whatever they want to call it. If she doesn't, get a new one.

Keep your CLINICIANS in the loop.

The clinical staff at healthcare organizations come and go frequently throughout the day from their clinic, other facilities, teaching obligations, and a variety of shifts. There is a strong possibility that some missed the leadership retreat held yesterday or the standing meeting on their scheduled day off. Some may have easily missed a lot of memos and discussions about new directives, initiatives, tech implementations; the list goes on.

      Nurture the professional relationships that exist in your organization, with plenty of face time and personal contact. Round at random times throughout the day and week, including weekends and nights. Post a daily, running blog or journal for internal staff and partners, with outcomes of daily events and meeting minutes, to keep everyone up to date on the state of the organization.

Healthcare has multiple PERSONALITIES.

Visit your staff and departments at random hours of the day, on odd days, holidays, the hectic days and quiet ones.

Visit unannounced.

Come bearing gifts.

Find out if there really are ghosts on this floor on Sunday evenings. Find out how these services get along so well at night but struggle during the day.

Does everyone know you? Do you know them?

Make it a point to find out the many faces of your organization by visiting them in their element.

Just because they are GOOD at what they do . . .

. . . doesn't mean they can manage.

When you think about promoting star clinicians or staff to a management position, always consider the Peter Principle: you don't want to promote them to their level of incompetence. Just because he's an excellent nurse doesn't mean he can manage the department. He's always going to be more valuable to you as a nurse.

Don't promote your staff to positions beyond their capabilities or interests and goals. You aren't doing anyone any favors.

But when you do, make sure to teach new managers how to manage, how to lead, to share, and to communicate. It's much more than a power trip or a pay raise.

SPONSOR, don't just mentor, your rising stars.

It isn't enough to mentor or coach those who report to or work for you. For true career growth and opportunity, leaders need to sponsor their rising stars, to open doors, invite them onto the next level, encourage their initiative and increasing levels of responsibility, and introduce them to the people and resources that will be part of their future.

Don't begrudge them their success and next steps. Someone did it for you.

C-suite: Leaders or PRIMA DONNAS?

It usually takes a lot of training, experience and ambition to rise to the top of an organization. Not everyone does it well once they arrive.

The C-suite needs to reflect the drive, focus, and the mission of the organization. It can't be afraid of hard work, dirty work, innovation, and teamwork.

And it must never be just about the paycheck. Everyone will know if it is.

> *The bottleneck is at the top of the bottle. Where are you likely to find people with the least diversity of experience, the largest investment in the past, and the greatest reverence for industry dogma?*
> *At the top.*
> Gary Hamel, Strategy as Revolution / HBR 1996

Make meetings MEANINGFUL.

Endless meetings, meaningless meetings, the wrong attendees, late-arrivers, weak agenda, smart-phone surfing, off-site training sessions for the masses, poorly prepared presentations (PowerPoint — *still?*).

Meetings can be huge time-wasters. Make them more meaningful.

Meetings, when they are needed, are successful only when the group is right. Who's included and why? Is membership representative of the key roles needed to accomplish its goals? Or does it resemble a high school party when the parents are out of town, and everyone and their Facebook friends show up?

Deciding on the participants of any committee or meeting is just like building a board of directors: each member has a distinct role, a responsibility to actively contribute, to bring and deliver feedback from their constituency, and a goal to make the outcome meaningful. All meetings are working meetings.

Always have an agenda. Send it out in advance, electronically.

Retire meetings and committees that have lost any semblance of meaning or accomplishment.

Start meetings at 5 or 10 minutes after the hour. You're less likely to have stragglers. You can jump right into the agenda. A meaningful meeting allows for transit between other meetings, time to respond to calls or messages, and other work commitments. It anticipates the inevitable post-meeting, frequently most creative, hallway chat. Really good ideas are generated in hallways.

And most importantly, starting a few minutes later gives everyone a chance for personal time without worrying about being late.

Now that your meeting has begun: Respect your audience. Never, repeat: never reinforce anyone's tardiness by reviewing what s/he missed.

Added bonus: End your meeting early. Set aside 5 to 10 minutes at the end of every agenda for comments, questions, or to simply adjourn and catch the next meeting...the one that might unfortunately start exactly on the hour.

Thanks. Meeting adjourned.

The Board of Directors must LOOK like its market.

The healthcare market is primarily female and middle-class. They are your guests, patients, staff, healthcare decision-makers. You know that.

A board that looks like its market is the only board that can point you in the right direction that the organization needs to go for long-term excellence and success.

Now, to represent your market in the best way you can, increase the number of middle-class females on your board to make up the majority, and give them the space, the opportunity, and a safe environment to use their voice for your organization.

TRAIN your Board.

Give them homework. Expect them to contribute their expertise, community insight and opinions. Let them help leverage their talents to build your organization.

Ask them for specific feedback, to seek and deliver the information you need to better run your hospital, clinic or organization.

Your board is your eyes and ears on the community, access to your current and potential benefactors, to your patients, customers and business and community trends. It can provide invaluable insight and intelligence about - you!

Train them to do their job for the benefit of their organization.

Beware the
PERKS of the office.

You've worked hard, climbed the ladder and you've finally arrived at the top. The work is hard, the perks are impressive, but the message you send will be tricky if you want an engaged and committed staff.

For crying out loud: never empty the executive suite to attend the same seminars, conferences, or industry meetings at luxury resorts. The message you send to your staff (who doubtless received a minimal wage increase along with a reduced departmental education budget) is that the rules don't apply. They will see a disconnect between the mission and leadership commitment to it.

When an annual conference or seminar beckons, send an executive representative and one or two new leaders. When they return, they'll get to share and pass along their newfound knowledge to the leadership teams who remained behind to run the ship.

Lessons learned? You've demonstrated that your responsibility is to your staff, to the organization. And when you can pass on what you know, you've truly learned something new.

People who lead people are the LUCKIEST people in the world.

Leadership is about creating the future: creating an organization to serve the community, the patients and guests, and all of those who are coming up behind.

Preparing the organization for the future is a noble task, growing future leaders a humble task, and the best leaders understand that.

You will move on, you are dispensable, after all, but that's not a bad thing: You get to grow your people for the future.

Leave a shining mark.

Everything needs a CHAMPION.

Initiatives, projects, goals, technology, innovations or improvements - every new or existing and ongoing project needs an executive owner.

Especially important to the success of innovations are those executives who have the ability to work magic with bureaucratic processes and roadblocks. But not one who is a bureaucrat herself.

Offer up your time and support to get innovations off the ground, and to give best practices a fresh look and commitment. Communicate your commitment and follow through.

Then do it, and stick with it.

ATTEND staff and department meetings.

Set aside time and commit to attending your staff's department meetings on a periodic basis. Let your staff know who you are, that you are there, accessible, and listening to them. Remind them that you want and need their help to move the organization in the direction of excellence.

Listen to everyone's concerns, their problems, and their complaints. Listen; don't monopolize the meeting.

And especially, learn about their ideas, their hopes and wisdom. Here's a chance to see how your organization really operates.

CONSULTANTS.
Or, who's running the ship?

Healthcare consultants are everywhere, and their numbers seem to grow daily. They can often provide a distinct and neutral one-time function to improve your organization, or fill in when leadership is short-staffed. It's not uncommon, though, for healthcare organizations to rely on consultants to provide the skills the leadership team should already be paid to possess.

Before you spend large sums on outside services, recognize: Why you need them, What they will provide that you are not already paying someone a salary to do, Who the best expert is for your organization's needs and budget, How they plan to accomplish the task and integrate it into the whole, and When it can be completed without them needing to up-sell to complete the task.

Then make sure it happens and they move on, not in.

Employee CONCERNS and complaints are not a curse.

Employee complaints may be an annoyance, but it's best to pay attention. Don't wait for the results of exit interviews to learn about the issues raised by your staff. It's a bit late for those you've invested in and lost, and your reputation is on the line at that point.

It's much easier and quicker to respond to employee concerns and complaints when they are still small and haven't had time to germinate; kudzu is next to impossible to remove.

So, whatever the issue is, big or seemingly small, give it at least some consideration. Create an employee council to review complaints, to present a peer-based evaluation and solution resource for staff concerns. Like building trust and respect, do something about it.

4
Mission & Vision

The POWER of an effective mission statement.

An organization's mission statement helps its leadership, staff and all of its customers envision a direction, a big picture and a purpose. Does yours?

A solid yet simple (not simplistic) mission statement gives a group a common language to help identify their work. It can transcend internal conflict and seemingly petty concerns of the moment. It can pave the way to building trust, confidence and movement in the direction the organization's leaders are aiming toward.

Try creating a simple mission statement, with fewer than 10 words. You might try to add a power statement: one or two words that evoke action: Right Care. We Care. First Stop. These are easy to remember and easy to instill in every staff member's engagement, training, and message.

Every system is perfectly designed to get the RESULTS it gets.

Paul Batalden MD

    Whether it's your relationship with your guests and patients, your community partners, your payers, regulators, clinical and physician colleagues, service lines and resources, or the staff—your healthcare organization will function exactly as you set it up and allow it to function.

    Set in motion the system you want, the excellent organization you want it to create to care for you when you need it. A solid mission and goals, staff with exceptional clinical skills, processes that don't get bogged down in bureaucracy, and a culture of innovation that can build and renew quality and safety quickly and effectively.

    Be the change, as they say.

SUNLIGHT is the perfect antiseptic.

Whether it's the public hospital's financial status, a physician's malpractice record, or the HospitalCompare report, transparency is good; it's cleansing.

Errors can happen to anyone, anywhere and at any time. Do everything possible to eliminate them. But don't bury your mistakes. Just as sunlight is a good antiseptic, so is transparency. It can, and often does, hurt a bit, sometimes a lot. But it also opens up the chance to improve what needs improving, whether it's clinical care or financial standing; to dare the competition to be better; and to hold healthcare accountable for its safe and effective patient care, its costs and quality.

Transparency can start big, important, and rewarding conversations, and it's good for business.

Environmental services and critical care are in the SAME business.

In healthcare, everyone's job is about taking care of one another, the customers, guests, patients, and staff. No one in the hospital can do it alone, no one is above it all, and everyone should be doing it for the same reason. Respect that, teach and build that, and acknowledge it.

Is your business in the RIGHT business?

Is your organization a hospital, a health system, a multi-specialty clinic, or is it really something else? When you understand your core competencies, your mission, your market, and your community's needs, you will have a clue about who you are and where you ought to be right now.

Being an excellent, second-to-none multi-specialty care clinic is a far better place to be in the world than a second rate, mediocre hospital with hit and miss safety and quality, unreliable safety and a poor reputation.

The PERFECT is the enemy of the good. Voltaire

It's too easy to let the perfect, the great, be your goal. You can hope for and wait around for accurate data, 100% buy-in, perfect procedures, or the best time to prove a point or take action. How long will that take? Does the perfect ever happen, really?

It's often better to take advantage of small, quick trials, a critical mass, or a lull in the conversation. See what happens, seek out tribal knowledge, and go with best hunches.

Be productive and embrace trial and error, learning from your small mistakes to learn and then continue moving onto bigger discoveries.

We're #1. Now what?

Fantastic!

Now you get to do it all again for the rest of the day, and tomorrow. And this time, do it a bit better.

Mature your core, your processes. Create a patina, an environment that is wise, well tended and trustworthy.

Keep your PRIORITIES clear.

First, do no harm. Keep your patients, staff and everyone you encounter at your organization safe from harm, mistakes, and fear.

Embrace your common core, what you know you do best, and do best consistently.

The loudest voice isn't always the most important. There are lots of loud, bossy voices in healthcare. Most are not important, just needy. Listen to the most important voices.

Suspect bright shiny objects for what they are: shiny. Beware of the new and cool stuff. Keep your priorities clear.

Embrace your institution's MEMORIES.

Healthcare trends go in cycles, and lessons can be learned from those who have been there and done that over the years.

Tap into the experiences of employees, donors, board members, and others who have been with your organization for a while. Learn how the organization's culture has evolved, how it's handled the changes and challenges, its evolving relationships and partnerships.

Institutional memories can give you insight into quick start opportunities or help you recognize the signs that, maybe, it's best to go slow.

KNOW who you are.

Every organization tells a story, whether it's official or not, just like a person's sense of style tells theirs: casual, diplomatic, sloppy, excellent. It establishes your reputation, the bias behind comments people tell about you. Maybe your organization is telling the world it is trustworthy; it's the only game in town so deal with it; or it's little but exceptional: the Little Engine that could. Is this the story you want, or have your customers created a different one for you?

It's important that everyone in your organization can tell, live and believe the same story, with a theme that runs through each and every encounter, service, product and commitment. Food services and critical care should use the same narrative to connect to their customers and guests.

RECOGNIZE your strengths and weaknesses.

Your organization's goals and plans must be built on reality.

Don't waste time and money planning to build a bigger version of programs that don't work or that continue to fail, or on services that are out of reach for your resources, or on programs that are unnecessary to meet the needs of your unique market.

Improve what doesn't work. Make them better before you create anything new.

Focus your energies and resources on what you do best. Then do them the best.

Make excellence your PRIORITY or don't waste your time.

Do you chip away at performance projects with a little bit of energy, letting distractions take over? Do you begrudge excellence pursuits the time, money and oversight they deserve to see them through?

If the big picture is excellence, then commit to it.

Otherwise, don't waste everyone's time. You either want it or you don't. Just buckle down and do your work.

VOLUNTEERS are also the face of your organization.

If your organization has a volunteer staff, set up a rigorous recruiting and training program, and recognize and retain them just as you would your paid staff.

It's definitely okay to hold your volunteers accountable for what they do. They are just as much a part of the organization as everyone else. And like everyone else, once trained, you don't want to lose them.

Publish an ANNUAL report.

An Annual Report is a report card of sorts, a summary of your organization's performance, its personality, and hopes for the future. Chances are, it might look and sound great; but even if it reveals mediocre performance, at least you know.

Like all report cards, especially the better ones, an Annual Report gives you strategic information and direction, direction where improvements need to be made, and what strengths can be pursued.

Your Annual Report tells your community about one of its most valuable resources. It can be reassuring, informative, enlightening, as well as a call to action.

SHARE data early and often.

Sharing your data, especially with cross-functional and internal teams and programs, will help you get the best information and build the best services you are looking for. While you run the risk of exposing the skeletons in the closet, you encourage fresh eyes to see what exists. Share data early, while the protocol are being built. It will limit defensiveness.

Openness with your data shines a light on the need for better clinical documentation, for a technological upgrade, or maybe a stronger skill set in the data lab.

Invest in INNOVATION.

Healthcare can change on a dime. New tech, procedures, treatment processes. The best way to handle it is with an atmosphere that embraces improvement and innovation.

Designate at least a non-negotiable 1% of your budget to innovation and skunk-works efforts. Encourage your staff to bring their best stuff to the table to improve the performance and care at your organization.

By encouraging user-generated innovation, you are guaranteed a higher level of staff engagement, ownership and that elusive stickiness everyone wants and has trouble finding. Invest in both the resources and culture of innovation and stickiness will follow.

What does your organization want to be when it GROWS up?

In a perfect world, what would your organization be like? There's not much you can do about CMS regulations, HEDIS questions, and Joint Commission standards, so why not beat them at their own game: set the bar higher and wider.

Hold your clinicians to world-class standards. Every one of them would relish the connection to a world-class organization.

Make ethical standards central to everyone's performance.

Reinvent the cafeteria as a 5-Star restaurant.

Invest in your dream now by cultivating innovation, best and evidenced-based practices, human-centered design, open and over-communication.

And whatever you do, make it meaningful for the long haul.

Self-pay PATIENTS.

Build high quality, lean and mean care processes into your system to add value for all of your customers. It improves your efficiency for everyone, especially your self-pay and charity care markets.

Self-pay patients will learn to recognize your efforts to provide the best quality and value for their money. They become better-informed patients, treating their healthcare as any reasonably informed, price and value conscious customer does. But remember, there are limits to what they will know, unless they venture on to medical or nursing school training.

Become a kinder, gentler, and thankful organization, and your market may learn not to begrudge your efforts to collect.

CHARITY care.

Healthcare is virtually unaffordable for the average person who doesn't have health insurance. Every healthcare organization, from hospital to clinic, will encounter the need to provide charity care to a segment of their market at some time.

Build compassionate care into your brand and delivery model. Develop a network of care that promotes preventive as well as chronic care services, with a focus on the least expensive or resource intensive options.

Charity care doesn't mean you have to give away the farm. But don't begrudge it - ever. Never dump your patients. That's always bad karma.

5
Quality

Standard is not GOOD enough.

A 'D' grade is a bad grade; kids all over the country get punished for bringing home a 'D' on their report card.

But it's still a passing grade.

How does that 'D' grade look on your patient safety outcomes, HEDIS, CMS and Joint Commission evaluations, or your annual report?

You don't have to perform like the bottom half of the class. It does take leadership with a strong will, commitment to quality goals, best practice oversight, clinical and performance checklists, and willingness to nurture collaborative relationships throughout the organization.

Everyone has a chance to rise to the top of the class.

Standard just isn't good enough in healthcare.

LOST in a sea of data.

Most healthcare organizations have so much data they don't know what they have, where it is, how good it is, or how to use it. It's often locked away in silos, with trolls under bridges who won't let it out or share it without exhorting a high political price.

Create an environment that values access to and cross-functional sharing of data to solve many of your organization's performance, regulatory, and outcome issues. Get it out of the IT department and into the services that can use it.

How do they DO that?

The United States rarely scores in the Top 10 on any international scale of health outcomes, with the exception of the amount of money spent on healthcare.

For ideas to improve your organization's outcomes and to provide the best patient care you can, set your sights broader, on examples from around the world. From data keeping to best practice models of care, there is plenty to be shared. Look farther, internationally.

OUTSHINE the competition.

Don't follow the herd. Set the quality standard in your community, your state, even in the industry.

Define what it means to be the best.

SHARE best practices throughout.

Each of your organizational or clinical departments can struggle to discover its own key to success. Or, with good leadership and a safe environment, they can share what they know, their successes and best practices, and how they put it into action.

Encourage services to share their experiences and efforts to increase the chances that the whole organization will be able to move forward. Sharing best practices creates an environment of innovation and improvement, providing patient and staff care that will be second to none.

Make it easy to COMPLY.

Whether it's regulations, policies or patient care, simply make processes and procedures easier to comply, to not make mistakes.

Remove barriers to best care, improve clinical and customer training, remodel the environment of care with proper equipment if necessary, create safe environments to speak up, adopt checklists, add hard stops to documentation systems, and adopt best practices from other industries who have won the compliance battles.

Make it easier to the job right the first time.

Dashboards are TOOLS, not goals.

It is fashionable and practical to have dashboards to present your group's performance metrics in a simple, easy to read format. Often times, however, they are the goal, and the data they present are never used.

If you go down the dashboard road, learn how to develop simple yet effective tools with clear graphics and meaningful data that everyone can use to monitor performance and place in time.

First, learn how to identify and measure what's truly important to your audience. Then design dashboards with simplicity and clarity in mind.

You want only a few, and each one must be understandable in a nanosecond.

MORE isn't always better.

In healthcare, the STOP button isn't always considered to be an acceptable treatment option. For many reasons, whether it is to try the latest treatment, or the next big thing, or because it simply can be done and clinicians have the means, or when the patient or family insist, or whether it's simply to make more money. More isn't always better.

While the patient gets to make the final decision, you have to be the professional who advises the merits of care and the options. It's also responsible to advise when it is the best time to stop. You can advise that more won't necessarily be better.

When you've done what you can do, know when to stop.

BIOETHICS.

Healthcare providers need to always consider the notion that just because they can do something, it doesn't mean they should. Just because there is guaranteed payment, a new source of revenue, it doesn't mean you should do it.

Remove an asymptomatic tumor from the leg of a bedridden 95-year-old? Implant 8 fertilized eggs into an IVF patient? Good decisions, based on best-practice and good ethics? Think better.

Integrate a rigorous bioethics program and system of thought into every clinical and financial program discussion and interaction. Don't shy away from the hard questions. It's part of the quality of your organization.

You make it. You USE it.

Every leader of every hospital and healthcare organization must be required to use the services their place provides when they and their families need care.

If it's not safe enough, private enough, or high quality enough for the organization's leaders, then it's not good enough for anyone else either.

Make the acronyms and credentials COUNT.

Healthcare professionals are by tradition and training bound by credentials. But the alphabet soup following one's name can also be as much about show and promotion as substance.

One of the most trusted, widely respected and published physicians I know graduated from an Ivy League medical school but uses a ½-page resume, and he never uses his titles. His actions count.

Back up your alphabet soup with substance and performance. Truly talented people don't need the props.

TEST the data.

Garbage in = garbage out. When you are set up to capture the best data, your organization can feel confident that it's facts and intelligence will reinforce sound business decisions, improve patient care, create valuable clinical integration, and forge stronger relationships with clinical and business partners.

Run, test data queries often. And make sure they are reviewed with fresh and knowledgeable eyes to keep it meaningful.

Food services can be the HEART of your organization.

Food evokes feelings of caring, comfort, healing. Just like home, the hospital kitchen and food services can be where the heart of the organization lives. Hospital food for patients, staff and guests doesn't have to be bland, boring and wiggly to pass nutrition tests.

Welcome to 21st-Century gastronomy: local, fresh, diverse, and tah-dah: healthy. Hire a talented chef and nutritionist to create delicious menus and complementary sustainable practices. Open up innovative opportunities for human interaction and education, guest satisfaction, and social responsibility too. Create a company garden for fresh herbs and produce; a cafe look and feel to evoke a *third place* for your staff and guests. You can't lose.

As someone once said, it's not brain surgery, but it can help you do the brain surgery.

ETHICS:
personal, professional.

Are ethics only in the eye of the beholder? Compliance to regulations and laws to prevent missteps or legal entanglements can be managed and policed. But a culture of high integrity and personal and organizational ethics needs to be modeled and nurtured. It's what gives the regulations and laws their meaning and purpose.

A culture of ethics, where safety, quality and integrity are embraced, demands an organization's commitment to its value.

Set high standards, not easy shortcuts, for yourself, your leaders, and your staff.

Set clear expectations for yourself and everyone in your organization.

Walk the talk.

Low EXPECTATIONS.

Beware the Fundamental Attribution Error of the soft bigotry of low expectations. How sad it is for any company, but especially healthcare organizations, to settle for mediocrity or worse, whether it's the level of patient care, the quality and taste of the cafeteria food, or even the facility's landscaping and upkeep.

Set your standards high, and if it is a local issue, simply don't settle for low community norms if they exist. Raise the bar.

Promote SKILL development.

Your organization is like a small town in a high intensity industry: it's a culture within a culture. Small organization or large, your staff brings a variety of behaviors, training, and work habits to their jobs. That creates a lot of opportunity for variation in their interactions, performance, and the care delivered. Add clinical and business silos and you have an interesting mix of skills and abilities.

From the use of checklists to service standards requirements, establish consistent, best practice behaviors, service standards and actions. Build skill development resources to improve competencies and nurture an overall culture of excellence and patient experience.

Does the technology PLAY well together?

Medical device and technology vendors are everywhere these days, trying to sell the latest and greatest solutions, often to problems you never knew you had.

When you spy or need a new toy, make sure it plays well with what you already have and actively use.

Does the latest ED patient tracking technology talk with the inpatient EMR? Can you trace patient outcomes and other data wherever a patient travels within the system? Can clinical and financial data merge to give you a global picture and solid business intelligence?

Conduct due diligence with all vendors and contracts to keep your technology coordinated.

Include PAYERS in your marketing plans.

Take advantage of all the information your payer representatives gather from your organization, as well as all you can gather from them. From patient care and claims to reimbursement strategies, policies and product changes, pay attention to it all.

Your payers have data galore about your patients. Tap into its treasure trove of information. Your payers can loop you into marketing and business development resources to help you improve your organizational services, help you find gaps in your patient and referral access, and even enhance your clinical outcomes.

6
Safety

Listen for the CANARY in the coal mine.

Every organization has a canary, a telltale alarm that something's going wrong. Listen, and learn to trust what it's telling you; it will be a symptom of an underlying problem or a crisis ready to happen.

Increasing numbers of falls, stubborn infection rates, and high staff turnover are problems, definitely. They are also warning signs that your organization has fundamental problems somewhere, maybe with clinical skills, staffing, or leadership, a fundamental problem that needs to be addressed immediately.

Investigate the signs and symptoms, then dig deeper to find the real disease: Do unanswered call lights lead to increased falls? Do the medical staff neckties or fake fingernails relate to increasing infection rates? You might be surprised.

Hospitals can be the WORST place to be when you are trying to get well.

There is a lot of stuff going on in hospitals. They can transfuse and infuse, fix breaks and problems, remove trouble, repair traumas and fight serious illness. But hospitals are notoriously too bright, too noisy, too chaotic, too infectious, and often too inhuman a place for sick and hurting humans to recover.

The best place to be is the place that allows the most appropriate care with the right, most effective amount of care and comfort, and the least amount of disruption., at the right price

Set up a community of resources to provide your patients with the best, safest, effective, and highest quality care services and environments, in order to get the right care at the right time.

We LOVE safety regulations.

Why is it easier to get a restaurant shut down for failing to comply with food service standards than it is to shut down a hospital for failing to meet its safety and quality regulations?

Whether it's CMS regulations, Joint Commission accreditation, or clinical or insurance credentialing, regulations and standards are intended to keep healthcare services and organizations safe, and for demanding performance that meets quality benchmarks.

Regulations are the basic level, the first step, to keeping everyone, including the facility, functioning at their best. Regulations are designed to create an environment that keeps patients safe.

Everyone in healthcare, from clinicians to administration, is aware that regulations and best-practice standards are simply the 'Duh' way to practice.

So, everyone:

Wash your hands and use disinfectant gel or glove up with each patient. Do it publicly; in front of your patient is best.

Remove dirty booties, gowns and lab coats when you leave the surgical and clinical areas; clinicians should not wear long ties, scarves, or any clothing that hangs from your body when you treat patients; no hand and dangling arm jewelry; and long, and definitely no fake, fingernails.

Never begrudge the work of the CMS, Joint Commission, or other examiners, and welcome their critical eye to see what is doubtless commonplace and unseen to the staff.

Don't become defensive when they find problem areas. Learn from it, and fix what ails your organization.

Keep CALM and carry on.

Designate quiet areas for medication management and dispensing, ditto for medical charting.

Reduce noise. Limit overhead announcements to the most critical announcements. Too much noise becomes white noise and won't be heard. Too much noise stalls healing, reduces appetite, and increases stress and anxiety. Too much noise limits clear thinking.

Consolidate the clutter of e-devices, from multiple pagers, to cell and smart phones. Teach best cell phone practice to reduce distractions.

Teach conflict management and communication skills. Most importantly, create safe environments for staff to speak truth to power, to raise issues about safety and quality without fear of reprisal.

Heal your organization with calm.

Never excuse the INEXCUSABLE or the mediocre.

It could be your child on the wobbly gurney, in the loud, chaotic treatment room, alone on the cold bed, on the noisy unit, with the overbearing, stressed clinicians.

Are you still comfortable? Can you excuse the inexcusable now?

Make it SAFE by design.

All sound healthcare organizations, just like exceptional manufacturing plants and 5-star restaurants, anticipate and preempt the predictable problems inherent in their industry. Make your organization and its practices safe by design, not retrofitted by ongoing poor performance.

Regulatory compliance is an easy one to anticipate and design to. Even new regulations that come out each year are predictable. Pay attention.

Strong relationships with well-trained, exceptional clinicians will enhance your quality and safety, allowing important conversations and improvements when needed. Make care safe by design.

Attention to environmental hazards, architectural and facility best practices, anticipating and meeting guest and client needs and comfort, and exceeding expectations: Safe by design will help prevent mishaps and expose prime opportunities to improve staff ownership and empowerment.

If everything is STAT, nothing is stat.

Just like the boy who cried wolf, people will stop listening.

Clean WINDOWS =
clean operating rooms.

Perception is reality. If your guests see clean windows when they arrive at your facility, they will probably assume the rest of the place is clean, that it's sterile and safe and well taken care of.

Attention to the smallest details, the nooks and crannies, will also instill a mindset of excellence in your staff that will extend throughout the entire organization.

Your guests and patients will see it. They will feel it.

And guaranteed, clean windows will instill trust in your patients, guests and partners.

The PURPOSE of rules and regulations.

Recognize the reason for the vast rules and regulations in healthcare, and acknowledge what can happen when they are ignored. Like the recurring disasters in the mining, oil well drilling, nuclear energy, and food industries, healthcare Never Events and out of control infection rates and malpractice are just the beginning of the problems that happen in healthcare when regulations are discounted or ignored.

It's time healthcare emulated the airline industry: Not many plane crashes these days, are there?

Establish best practice models and develop checklists to identify the basic, critical steps to deliver care seamlessly and consistently. Make it easy to meet the rules and regulations. Let them become your foundation, so they won't trip you up.

Be the safe PLACE to work.

In the professionally silo-ed environment of healthcare, colleague rivalry, egos and turf struggles can challenge the most assertive staff, which can impact both employee and patient safety and care.

Does your staff feel safe to speak their mind when patient safety is compromised, trusted when they speak truth to power, empowered to challenge the culture for improvement and quality?

Does management have their back when they need to speak out on safety issues or inappropriate or abusive behavior?

Teach managers and leaders to listen, to be attentive, to pick up on the telltale signs of safety concerns, and to make solutions immediate, clear and widespread. Provide a safe and healthy environment for your employees to create a safe and healthy environment for your staff and your patients.

Good leaders are human SHIELDS.

Use your seniority for a good cause: run interference for your staff and employees. A good cause is especially those staff whose work requires sustained periods of concentration—nurses and other knowledge workers who need space and time for medication prep, documentation, decision-making, for example.

Unnecessary meetings, meddlesome superiors, bullying coworkers, staff shortages, unproductive downtime, distractions and time-sinks kill morale. More importantly, they can adversely impact patient care and safety.

Shield your important workers from activities that prevent them from doing their best work. That would probably mean most of them.

A good program with no COMPLIANCE—isn't.

The best program in the world, the one that has everyone at industry conferences saying, "let's do that at our place, too!" is so tempting. Great programs will work anywhere, won't they?

Not necessarily so.

As the work of many NGOs, aid and humanitarian efforts will attest, the most successful programs are always generated from the ground up, with grassroots, organic input right from the start. If it isn't authentic and personal to your audience, you'll struggle getting it off the ground and more to the point, to get it to stick.

Compliance won't happen until it sticks; until it's owned.

Before you start implementing a new initiative or program, listen to the people on the front line and find out what they know. They know a lot. Is everyone just waiting for the trainers to leave so they can get back to their real jobs, the way it was before?

Don't waste your time pushing on the door marked 'Pull.'

An ANGRY patient is valuable.

Just as you can learn more than you want to know from a crisis, you can learn a lot from your angry, unsatisfied patients and guests, probably more than from the happy ones.

The food has no flavor, or the nurse won't respond to the call light. Halls are too noisy, or the patient's doctor is standing just outside the room but hasn't visited in days. All problems that can be fixed.

Take some time to parse out the real story behind the complaint and fix what's broken. It's certain this isn't the first time that particular problem has ever occurred; this guest just had the need to let you know it was unacceptable.

Is there a CORRELATION between unanswered call lights and fall rates?

It's just a hunch.

It's a natural human instinct for people to want to be independent, to do things for ourselves, to remind ourselves, and others, that we are still competent and capable. So why is anyone surprised that, when the nurse won't answer the call light, but the patient really needs to use the bathroom, she will just try to make it there on her own?

Test the hunch. If your fall rates are high, every hunch is worth checking out.

Daily stand-ups create FOCUS.

Daily huddles, stand-ups or check-ins, are a valuable activity at the start of every shift, especially in large organizations. When run well, they can enhance the relationships of the group or department, reinforcing individual and collaborative responsibilities. They drive energy and attention to the moment as well as toward longer-term goals, and they guarantee the visibility of every member.

Establish rules of engagement and participation in daily stand-ups and commit to them. In healthcare, there's always something going on to report out. A safe staff environment demands presenting both the good and bad news. No one gets to hide, nor should they feel they need to.

Everyone participates. From birthday greetings to major never-event reporting, this is a hospital: there will be drama!

Shortcuts, workarounds, and JERRY-RIGGING.

Jerry-rigging is what a sailor does to fix something quickly in order to stay afloat. It's never meant to be permanent and is definitely not preferred to the quality standard.

When clinical or other work is performed infrequently, when standard, best practices haven't been taught or imprinted into muscle memory, or when stress levels are high, clinicians and staff can resort to ineffective and dangerous shortcuts. They resort to jerry-rigging.

To limit the need for jerry-rigging and shortcuts, strengthen skills. With the curse of small numbers, try to integrate staff by experience level and demonstrated best practice skills.

Give everyone the chance to gain exposure, expertise with the rare situations but critical skills. Provide the resources to practice and maximize their peak performance.

7
Improvement

Consultants don't get a pass on PERFORMANCE.

Negotiate consulting contracts like you would solid employment contracts, with the end product and performance in mind. Consultants are paid big money for the work they promise, the disruption they pose, and the time they spend doing it.

Hold them to their promise.

Manage consultant contracts diligently. Put someone in charge of each one, preferably someone working directly with the problem at hand. This guarantees a set of eyes to see the entire landscape being improved, not just one piece of it, and not just one of possibly many consulting gigs.

This gives them a chance to oversee delivery, too.

Value everyone's time and get your money's worth.

Nor can they work MIRACLES.

You can't expect outside consultants to work miracles, to deliver solutions that are impractical, or that ignore the limitations of your organization. Consultants can't change an organization that isn't willing, ready or capable of making the changes necessary for improvement.

Consultants can't be held accountable for making the impossible happen. Sure, they'll gladly offer miracles - they'll take your money, and even up-sell to get more of it. But they also have an industry reputation to uphold. It isn't in their best interest to fail or under-perform.

Before you contract with consulting groups to provide analysis, expertise, process, or technical improvements, make sure you know what your organization can and is willing to do with that expertise.

Hold yourself accountable for taking an active role in being willing and able to implement recommended solutions and processes.

Survey-mania: make it STOP.

Like many busy, intelligent people, you've become selective about the surveys you choose to participate in. If the company or surveyor is known for its innovation and unfailing attention to customer service, then, sure, by all means, bring it on, you'll help them keep up the good work.

But many surveys are just boring; they are out of the box look-alikes; are meaningless, will probably not be used, and you know will be a waste of your time.

Figure out where your surveys can get the biggest bang for your research buck, and do no more. Respect your customer's time and intelligence.

Focus instead on actually providing excellent care.

From staff to customer feedback, there are ingenious, simple and effective ways to learn what you probably already know, without a survey.

Besides, you'll still hear about it if you mess up.

CHECKLISTS.

If it's good enough for professional pilots, count us in!

From the environmental care team to materials management to the surgical suite—there is a place for checklists to streamline appropriate and necessary procedures and to focus everyone on the task at hand.

Checklists ensure consistency in process and service delivery, from the tools and resources, personnel and support, to the necessary steps required from beginning to end.

Checklists allow new teams to work together with the same goal in mind. They give patients the confidence to feel safe with the care they receive. Checklists provide innovation the solid foundation it needs for support.

Nursing = IT.

Nurses are now, and will continue to be, the most intensive users of your IT resources. They must be included as an integral part of the IT department.

When considering the technology resources you need or will need to update for your organization, the nursing staff must be your primary audience to review its potential, its effectiveness and its ultimate success.

Bring nursing, from active leader to frontline users, into all IT discussions and demonstrations at the very beginning, and include them throughout the due diligence, vetting, implementation and operational processes.

Get IT out of its CAVE.

Welcome IT into the mainstream.

Introduce the IT team to the end-user—all of the end-users. Make sure they interact directly with the variety of technology users right from the start, from the light-bulb stage through implementation to the inevitable upgrades. No healthcare organization whose mission is excellent patient care wants an ineffective, unusable and very expensive toy. One that only the IT team understands, manages, and maybe even rations.

Not unheard of in healthcare.

And in healthcare, clinicians must be made permanent members of the IT team. Clinicians know the workflow, the terminology, the need to integrate, or not, a variety of systems, why hard-stops are invaluable, and the inevitable roadblocks and limitations to new processes.

Improvement is a MARATHON, not a sprint.

Six Sigma, Lean, Studer, Malcolm Baldrige, IHI. The list of improvement initiatives and consulting solutions goes on and on.

Improvement processes all work. They all lead to success.

Pick one. Stick to it. Commit to the long term. Improvement is a marathon, not a sprint. It is a long, sometimes tedious, process.

Find an improvement process that fits your organization's cultural, intellectual and clinical style, its needs and goals. Stick with it, for long-term and sustained improvement.

> *People tend to overestimate the short-term effects of anything while underestimating the long-term impact of everything.*
> openDemocracy

Don't get stuck at CRITIQUING.

Improvement processes don't need 100% buy-in just to be tested. Nor does the process need to be evaluated at every step of the way. Just like writing a paper: save the edits for the end.

Try the process out small, test with baby steps. Measure the outcome; see if there is any change. If you like what you see, roll it out to an ever-broader audience. Repeat.

Rapid-cycle testing, quick-starts, is one way to test innovation and improvement processes. It gets you over the critiquing stage, and on to the just do it, fun part. The delivery.

Watch out for those bright, SHINY OBJECTS.

There are always going to be new ways to do an old process, a new thing on the horizon that is guaranteed to bring quick results. Just like a new weight loss or exercise plan, a new and improved fix.

Innovation and improvement doesn't always need to involve bringing in the next great consultant or process, however. Often, the best, most creative solutions are often simply reworking what's already under your nose.

Remember that your organization and its vision are set up to deliver over the long haul; resist the bright, shiny objects and solutions unless they can truly add value, energy, and demonstrable change, and will seamlessly match your goals and brand.

Start small. Grow SMART.

Implementing improvement processes, starting new services, or bringing in consulting gigs are big and disruptive steps. Doing so without first developing and communicating a strategic plan or a few basic goals is bound to create unnecessary chaos and pushback. It is bound to set up an atmosphere of resistance and defensiveness, especially when you decide to do the really big stuff.

Set the stage for your initiatives by starting small, recruiting converts and champions, those early adaptors who will be the cheerleaders for your project.

And: Always under-promise and over-deliver.

Healthcare reform is an open invitation to BEST practices.

Healthcare reform, Accountable Care Organization, Medical Home, bundled payment mechanisms, RAC and other industry issues are perfect opportunities to establish innovative and evidence-based best practices and relationships in your continuum of care.

Instead of thinking of these issues as intrusive and more regulatory bumps in the road, think of them as chances to innovate; an opportunity to provide excellent, coordinated patient care; as strategies to address financial efficiencies; to drive best and evidence based clinical practices throughout the system.

Worst-case scenario: you can blame your way to newfound excellence on someone else.

Improvement projects cannot exist in a VACUUM.

Performance and service improvement projects will impact your entire system in one way or another.

When you are planning an improvement project, don't forget to coordinate your activities with others in the organization, whether they seem to be related or not.

Discuss new projects in executive team, board, planning, and management meetings, to give colleagues a chance to learn about what's going on, to share with their peers and others in the organization, and to pass the word to their groups for feedback.

Turning over stones you wouldn't normally consider may actually magnify the positive effect and reach of your new project. It can improve acceptance, lessen the resistance, and possibly grow an offshoot innovative project throughout the organization.

Keep your goals simple and FEW.

If your mission statement is longer than 10 words, it's too long.

No one can be all things to all people; don't try to be. Nor do you need to save the world on the first try—that takes a lifetime of baby steps.

Take the baby steps.

Likewise, if your strategic plan involves more than 5 goals, you have way too much going on for your organization to handle. Too much and you can't get everyone engaged to accomplish them *and* do their own basic work as well.

Start simply and basic, and establish easy processes to achieve your first few goals. When these have been met, and only when they become part of everyone's muscle memory, can you feel comfortable adding one or two new goals.

Business development RESOURCES abound.

Spread the business intelligence net wide. Use your data to learn what impacts your organization's service offerings, the shifts in your market, and the next steps you can take to fill in the gaps.

Demographics, technology, payment patterns, large employer trends, medical management, insurance and payer markets, clinical resources, economic changes, impact of natural and human disasters, epidemiologic trends. They can all affect your organization's effectiveness, its growth and relevance.

Tap every resource to uncover opportunities as well as constraints to your organization's success. Build them into your planning strategy.

To create change, make your INTENTIONS clear, specific, and possible.

In their nifty little book about change, *Switch*, Chip and Dan Health discuss three necessary components of change: emotion, logic, and a clear path for action. Check it out.

Every organization encounters the need and desire to change and grow. Change also comes with resistance. To ease the switch to the new, use clear and compelling directions, with motivations that meet both the emotional and rational needs of your organization. Create a clear, well-lighted path to get to there.

Reward the ENTREPRENEURIAL spirit.

Innovation doesn't come easy in this industry. Healthcare is built on status quo, researched clinical practices, checklists, and algorithms. But there's always room for improvement, especially with service and best practices. If you want excellence, reward the entrepreneurial spirit in your ranks.

Innovation takes imaginative minds, safe relationships, and a fertile, well-tended environment. It needs a place to think big thoughts and to operate like a nimble small business.

The results can be excellent patient care, rewarding business opportunities, improved revenue, clinical, patient, and staff satisfaction, more effective and appropriate care deliver. Innovation can engage staff and accelerate the improvement process, building success upon success.

Dare to take a few innovative steps and see what happens.

Bad artists copy.
Good artists steal.
Pablo Picasso

It isn't necessary to reinvent the wheel to build a good business or provide great service. If you've thought it, it's probably already been done. Beg, borrow, and steal.

Unless it's proprietary, tap into the successes, processes, business models, and examples of excellent healthcare organizations and services all around you. There is a lot of public data, research, and clinical process information to adopt and develop into your own.

And if you ask, people love to talk about their ideas and success stories. Invite them over for a brown-bag lunch to hear about their style and experiences.

Do you need a CONSULTANT for your consultant?

If you don't understand what your consultants are proposing, talking about, or actually doing for you, tell them. Hold them accountable for answering your questions so you and your staff get the full picture. You shouldn't need another consultant to help you figure out what your consultants are doing.

Every consulting group should provide an account or project manager to interact with you at not just the selling and contracting stage but throughout the implementation and sign-off level as well.

You need to be able to work with a single individual who will commit to, coordinate, and communicate with you about every service available to you for your needs. Don't settle for different individuals for each product. Don't settle for a product or an implementation you don't understand.

Embrace positive DEVIANCE.

Every organization and group has its little pods of excellence and innovation, services that shine, the rare teams that, simply and consistently, do it better than the others. They make the policies work better, beat the regulators at their own game, make patients and guests feel special, become the favorite service to work and partner with.

Let these folks out into the light to shine for everyone else who needs an example, a how-to or a kick in the pants.

INNOVATION: the last word to describe healthcare?

Unfortunately, it's true in too many ways.

Processes, procedures, hierarchies, silos, leadership, relationships, and physical environments become stale, habitual and blind to worst practices when innovation and improvement aren't recognized, valued, or shared. They become risk averse, entrenched in tradition.

Sadly, this stale, habitual, fearful, risk-averse and blind adherence to the status quo that is healthcare leads to lazy and contemptuous attention to safety and quality.

Fortunately, improvement techniques from the world of business and manufacturing are finding homes in healthcare: Crucial Conversations, 6-Sigma, Lean, Best Practices, Checklist initiatives, entrepreneurial vision.

You can also change that with a skunk-works team – a group focused on those ideas that can strike fear in the heart of the status quo.

Skunk-works is a place, virtual or bricks and mortar, where ideas and small changes can be imagined, vetted, tried on for size, tested and failed in safety, reworked and refined, and hopefully and eventually, scaled up for introduction to a wider audience.

Innovation and improvement can be scary endeavors but well worth the price when the organization experiences improved patient safety and outcomes (the ultimate goal), employee connection to their best work and colleagues, and contributions to the community at large.

What gets MEASURED gets managed.

This is an old truism. Whether it's the squeaky wheel, the trendy high revenue service line, or surgery start time outliers, that's where the leadership energy and resources will go.

Your commitment of time and resources needs to relate to your mission, to your organization's strategic goals. Otherwise, it is probably distracting you from the work you really hope to be doing. Those you've previously committed to will start to lose their focus and feel their work is unimportant or the goals you've created are just another pipe dream.

Make sure what you are measuring and spending your time on is where you want the organization's energy to go.

Tour your facilities
to find out what works
and what's BROKEN.

Take a tour around your hospital, its grounds and facilities, and rigorously check out the place. Then tour the competition - even check out places that provide other types of customer care and service, like high quality hotels, cafes and popular retail establishments.

Is there any reason your healthcare organization can't shine and perform like the places in your community that cater to the public, and deliver excellent care and service?

Discover ways you can help all your guests experience the best of your organization: Guest comfort means a warm acknowledgement, natural light and soft sounds, easy access to services, and confident and attentive staff. And the staff would value an excellent, ergonomic workplace.

The list is endless.

The VIEW from 10,000' always looks awesome.

Can you picture the iconic photo of Earth from the Apollo 8 spacecraft? The graceful blue and white globe rising over the moon, showing no trace of the wars and unrest on the ground. Simply beauty.

Like the beauty of the earth from space, the perceptions of a healthcare leader toward the value of improvement initiatives, the latest technology and clinical processes, the expensive remodel, may not always mirror their on-the-ground effectiveness.

New IT projects, reconstruction and other investments in improvement projects and change processes are astronomical and impact everyone. From the stratosphere, however, leadership bias can work overtime—for this much money, it had better all look great.

On the ground, it's not that simple. Systemic changes will always create chaos and havoc on the frontline. Vendors and consultants probably won't warn you about it, but they've seen it.

Be skeptical of the over-promise of the magic and effectiveness of major system overhauls. Keep your radar focused on what those on the ground tell you. Up close and personal, the details are menacing.

There is never too much good COMMUNICATION.

     Remember Communication 101 from freshman college: With every message, there is a sender and a receiver, and always, there will be…stuff…in…the,,,middle that distorts the message in some way. Add the so many, and counting, ways of sending and receiving messages, and there is just that…much…more…stuff…to get in the way of good communication.

     What to do?

     Over-communicate. Use a variety of strategic media and tools; make sure the receivers can and do receive your message; that the receivers know your expectations; make sure they have the skills and tools to follow-up or do whatever needs to be done with the message they receive. And repeat

*Everything that can be counted
does not necessarily count;
everything that counts
cannot necessarily be counted.*
Albert Einstein

The color of the walls in the patient rooms really counts. Really.

The amount of soap and disinfectant used annually by the hospital doesn't count as much.

Make what you count, count.

But never ignore the value of everything else that does.

Support the small BUSINESSES within.

Each service line and department in your hospital, clinic and organization can be treated as its own small business. Every one presents an opportunity to build its market, a brand within a brand, and generate a nifty revenue stream. Imaging, laboratory, infusion center, even the cafeteria, the list goes on; you are surrounded with a small business innovation lab.

Develop a laser focus to access the business intelligence resources hidden within your organization and make sure every manager and leader has immediate access to and training to be able to use this information.

With the support of innovative leaders, the budding entrepreneurs in your organization can create the true centers of excellence, the next Starbucks, of your organization.

8
Design

Recognize the AMBIENCE of your facilities.

Color, light, energy, mood, fresh air, sound, smells: each of these elements play an important role in the quality of care delivered and received, in your employee's moods, your colleague's interactions, even patient recovery.

If your goal is to deliver patient care that is safe and exceptional, you know that it's hard to heal or even to work in an environment that comes right out of Dickens or could double as a warehouse. The days of disregarding the ambience of the environment have gratefully been replaced. The multi-bed patient rooms and wards are gone; ditto the foul odors, green paint, noise, too much artificial lighting.

Design your facilities to capture the life, health, wellness, and emotion you want to provide.

Design with the HUMANS in mind.

Hospitals and healthcare organizations are built for human care but often are not designed for the humans who want to perform their best or need to heal and thrive.

Spaces of calm and order are needed for exchanging patient information at shift change and handoff, updating charts and dispensing medication. Designate 'Do Not Disturb' sections in every nursing area. Something as simple as a bright color change in a nook might do the trick.

Patient healing and recovery demand spaces of comfort, calm, privacy and human connection. It is especially critical when high tech is the norm, when stress is on high alert. Add soft surroundings, warm blankets, install comfortable lighting, reduce noise, and create quiet soothing sound.

Design with the humans in mind.

Have FRESH eyes.

Familiarity can breed contempt and blindness: broken equipment, out-of-date supplies, or no concierge at night are simply unacceptable in a best in class healthcare organization.

It shouldn't take a CMS surveyor to discover dirty or bloody linens lying around, or candy and coffee cups in the anesthesia carts. A handicap accessible public bathroom whose auto-door doesn't work, or an elevator lift that a person can't operate alone are not just nuisances. These are examples of broken equipment and simply need to be fixed.

Whether you hire a Secret Shopper or use a checklist on your daily rounds, start paying attention to the way things are in your environment. It will lead everyone to start paying attention and calling for fixes, too.

The look and feel of EXCELLENCE.

The aesthetics of the buildings and facility, their physical environment, and the relationship to the neighborhood speak volumes about your organization. It is your fundamental, public message of quality and care.

From outside to inside, the landscaping, color, texture, lighting, and cleanliness—it's all-important to your patients and guests in creating a welcome, safe place to receive care and to heal.

The look and feel of your place are equally important to your staff. It's critical to your overall success to create a work environment that honors and welcomes them, and respects their own need for compassion and well-being.

Watch the CLUTTER.

Too many initiatives. Stick with the best few, long term.

Too many consultants. Tap into in-house experts.

Too many vendors. Consolidate.

Too many insurance denials. Smooth out the admit process.

Too much noise. Speak with calm, soft confidence.

Too many goals. Simplify.

Too much unsupported tech. Due diligence.

Too much drama. Stop enabling.

Too many expired supplies. Clean out the main supply closet.

Too few follow-ups. Reward performance.

Too many forgotten staff birthdays and anniversaries. Inexcusable.

Too many ER visitors leave without being seen. Set up an urgent care center.

Too much data untouched. Give it a good home.

Design is CULTURAL.

Design is local.

You can't outsource the look and feel of your organization with an expensive architect or design guru, or the latest style from the coast. What works in Miami probably won't last long in Dayton.

Design is part of the culture. It looks and feels like home; it belongs. Involve everyone, from your staff to your community, in all building, space and environmental design efforts, from remodeling to new facility architectural design.

Design is and has to be organic, created and built from the local ground up. That's what excellent organizations do.

Design people spaces for respite and periodic ESCAPE.

Many experiences in healthcare are intense and dehumanizing. High-tech equipment, low-touch procedures, hard and cold surfaces, harsh lighting, unfamiliar terminology, and thoughts of unknown and frightening outcomes—they all work together to create an uncomfortable and stressful environment for patients and staff alike.

Create areas for patients and staff to decompress, spaces for quiet and calm, with soft surroundings, live plants that promise fresh air, low noise, natural and soft lighting, and comfortable seating areas with space for privacy, escape, and time alone.

SIGNAGE:
clear and simple.

Clear, simple, and above all, minimal, signage is essential to getting your guests and patients quickly and safely through the hallways of your facility.

Excellent signage is fundamental to patient and guest satisfaction, to operational and process efficiencies. It tells your world that your organization works.

If temporary signs, post-its, and random papers and posters are taped up and cluttering walls or tacked up to clarify directions or instructions, it's time to stop and begin again: it means your signage isn't working.

Do it right the first time. And don't depend on staff or others who are overly familiar with the place to evaluate its effectiveness. Use fresh eyes. And be merciless.

Airport terminal SEATING must go.

It's hard to believe this is still the norm in many healthcare environments. Even the better airports got the memo that this arrangement has seen better days.

Remember the primary reason your guests and patients are in the waiting room: they don't feel well, or they hope to stay well. Guests and patients need a bit of personal space, room to lie down or spread out if they feel too ill to sit, or space for the kids to wiggle and move (and they will, so don't expect them not to). Create spaces for families and their private conversations; subtle but distinctly separate areas for those with highly contagious illnesses.

With a bit of imagination and forethought, your waiting and guest areas can become exceptional little islands of tranquility and care. You will be be step closer to providing excellent healthcare.

Curb APPEAL matters.

Real estate agents have it right: Curb appeal sells.

Aesthetics are all about humans creating environments that help or improve the lives of other humans, often in profound ways, and in ways that are quite small and go unnoticed. It takes just a nanosecond, one of those moments of truth, to sum up an environment, and it makes an impression, for better or worse.

Don't worry about it trivializing your clinical work. Quite the contrary - it will only enhance what you do.

The nooks and crannies: the untended plants, overflowing garbage cans, discolored paint and unkempt grounds; those pesky, innocuous details that contribute to an unpleasant, even devastating experience for everyone, can undo the best clinical care you want to advertise.

Replace the creepy motel, utility company feeling with a well-tended, up-to-date, environment.

Make it look and feel better.

Design for all of the human SENSES.

Sight, sound, touch, smell, and taste are the five recognized human senses. Human-centered environments are built around them in basic ways, and excellent organizations go out of the way to focus on them.

In designing your facilities and environments for healing and wellbeing, remember that other senses such as temperature, energy and activity levels, pain, and balance need to be recognized and accommodated as well, to meet the heightened and sensitive needs of ill, anxious, sensitive, and hyperaware patients, guests and staff.

9
Market

Your INTERNAL customers are your primary customers.

No, it's not opposite day.

Your internal customers, from the frontline concierge and valet to the neurosurgeon and head nurse are your patient's caregivers. They are the ones who deliver the goods, who represent the best you have to offer. Your internal customer deserves a supportive, efficient, safe, and high quality work environment.

Are your patients and guests going to get the best care in the world if their caregiver is fearful, disrespected, uncared for, or disengaged from their work?

Happy, cared-for workers deliver.

> *A company is stronger if it is bound by love rather than by fear... If the employees come first, then they're happy.*
> Herb Kelleher, Southwest Airlines

The Emergency Department is a GOLDMINE of business opportunities.

Whether it's urgent care aimed specifically at the elderly, responding to community behavioral health needs, or addressing chronic disease management, the ED is an on-site idea and innovation incubator.

When not in emergency mode, the ED has data and resources to identify and create alternative high quality outpatient and outreach programs to meet non-emergent patient care and physician needs.

Tap into the data and see what's there. Innovate.

Change HAPPENS in spite of your plans.

As John Lennon sang, "Life is what happens when you're busy making other plans..."

All the strategic plans and goals in the world won't stop change from happening. You won't always know exactly what it will be, but you can anticipate it by building access to a system of resources, support, flexibility, and most important of all, a resilient and creative mindset that all change demands.

Just like the design of the Internet or Interstate highways, you can build your system's processes with alternative (escape) routes and pathways to adapt to or rapidly recover from the changes that are inevitable.

Mind the GAPS!

Know where the service and access gaps exist in your service environment, in your community, as well as in your market. These are the opportunities to build both your market and your patient care access.

Robust research and data gathering from the community, including from public resources, partners, payers, and consulting groups, can help identify obvious service, access, and resource gaps.

From healthcare provider access to technology tools, to current and proposed payment shifts; epidemiology by market sector, chronic disease management programs, and established partnerships—improvement opportunities can be found to impact your healthcare community and bring fresh and innovative strategies.

Think like a SMALL business owner for growth and excellence.

For improvement, strategic growth, creativity, and overall business excellence, it pays to think like a small company out to create and make money, not like a miserly penny-pincher that can survive by getting by.

Think like a small business owner to recognize the value of creating an image and spending money the right way in order to make money on the right opportunities.

You need to spend on innovation, marketing, and business intelligence. You don't need to spend an obscene amount, but enough, and wisely.

Decrease costs (Never Events, readmits); increase revenue (care coordination); increase value (chronic care management); improve quality (environment of care); and increase innovation (continuum of care).

The return will show and speak for itself in enhanced services, quality and improved business relationships and customer satisfaction.

Deliver value to your patient MIX.

Capture the demographic and clinical data on your emergency and acute care patient population to create the ideal blend of services with the most appropriate sources to meet their needs.

A population of elderly patients provides an opportunity to focus inpatient services on chronic care needs, fall prevention, hospital-induced dementia care, and mobility resources, as well as outpatient services from prevention screening to chronic disease management.

Maternity patients offer a chance to capture an entire family's care needs back in the community, including online wellness, health education, immunizations, and medical record keeping tools.

Orthopedic and elective markets afford an opening to an array of services in rehabilitation, sports medicine, prevention, wellness and lifestyle health management resources.

NURTURE your thought-leaders.

Cultivate the experts and thought-leaders within your organization and among your partners. They can become a valuable resource that will lend credibility to your organization. Whether it's community fundraising or securing a national grant, both your clinical and non-clinical experts are an indispensable resource to help you build quality and gain exposure.

Align your thought-leaders and experts with key audiences and use them effectively, both internally and out in the community. Nurture a stable of experts to provide expertise on a variety of topics and issues.

Create a TOOLCHEST of marketing resources.

Once you've established a strong image, a brand identity, and built exceptional core services, develop value-added resources for your customers, from patients and guests to your professional colleagues, partners and staff.

Health, wellness, and clinical online and in-house resources, can include health literacy tips and advice, exercise, weight loss, or disease management tracking tools, and access to clinical advice and referral services.

Professional resources can be specific to a physician's practice, patients and community demographics, or consultation services; a secure database for clinical care and disease management opportunities; and access to personal and clinical performance dashboards.

Focus on the simple solutions and opportunities. Make access easy and meaningful.

Know your AUDIENCE.

It's everyone who knows you. There's no escaping it.

Your current, past and future patients and their families, your employees, the neighborhood, your clinical partners and competitors, vendors, consultants, government regulators, politicians, extended family, the guy in front of you at the grocery store.

Remember, it's always showtime.

Know your customer.
SHE is you.

In the healthcare industry, like most every other, your customer is female.

She is your leadership, your staff. She is your patients, guests, internal and external partners, boards and vendors. She is your audience, your focus, the decision maker, your best customer and also your worst nightmare if you don't do it right.

From your clinical and service innovations, resources, environments, touch and feel, brand and messaging: create and build them all with her in mind.

Build your board, committees and services with your customers at the top of mind.

Strengthen REMOTE partnerships and networks.

Tele-health, teleconferencing, electronic tools, remote and web-based access to clinical and subject matter experts: State of the art resources can remarkably improve your ability to reach out to your remote, rural and isolated and demanding community partners, patients, and customers.

Whether it's cloud-based applications to the growing variety of technological tools available, utilizing the right, most appropriate and strategic resources can provide a value-added service to everyone in your network, improving access, care and efficiency.

And it's ecologically sound, too!

Start small, recruit clinical champions and move into the 21st Century world of healthcare.

10
Clinical Care

Embrace the CRISIS.

A crisis, the worst that can happen, is waiting to tell you something. When the crisis has been successfully resolved, it's a matchless opportunity to discover how well your place really works, what can and will eventually go wrong when you don't pay attention to details, and how you can prepare for the unexpected emergency.

A crisis removes the mask; it opens up new arenas for insight, growth, relationships, and it grants permission for improvement.

Take off the band-aids, the jerry-rigging, the non-essentials that get in the way of the good. Remove the sticky note reminders in charts and on the wall, on protocols. Bring in the right partners and staff.

Fix things the right way this time, so there is no crisis next time.

Be a CLINICIAN.

How easy is it to get a patient admitted to your facility or services? What makes it seamless or bumpy? Are there bottlenecks that can be removed? Are there excellent pathways to get your patient into and out of your facility when the time comes?

Do surgeries, procedures, and exams routinely arrive or start on time, when both you and the patient expect them to? How quickly and consistently can test and procedure results be available? Is support staff immediately available when needed for patient care?

Are patient records coordinated so their care is coordinated?

What are patients saying to you about this place? Why?

Look at your organization through the eyes of your clinicians; discover all the opportunities to build or integrate care processes throughout the system or organization, to improve both your professional life and especially, your patient care.

Understand WORKFLOWS.

Sounds simple. A clear appreciation and respect of the workflows can help you understand the constraints as well as opportunities to fix what might be broken and is holding back your organization's efforts to excel.

Are policies getting in the way of actually completing the work the best way possible? Are there too many, or maybe, simply, unnecessary, steps, roadblocks, or silos in the way of getting to the final goal? Is it as basic as inappropriate training, poor leadership, or staffing? Is it poor facility design? Hmm?

Figuring out the steps required to get from point A to Z, in the easiest, most efficient, effective and meaningful way will require input from those who actually do it. You need input from those who are personally invested in making it better. Improvement teams made up of representatives from every department that the workflow touches. That's a good start.

Policies must never OVERWHELM patient care.

If following policy leads to a 5-hour turnaround for pain medication orders, something's terribly wrong.

If following policy means patient checkout takes most of a day, something's wrong.

Fix what's broken. Always remember that the patient's wellbeing comes first. Replace policies if patients seem to be getting in their way.

Patient handoffs: think like a MASSEUSE.

If you've ever had a professional massage, you are familiar with the masseuse who barely breaks the physical connection with you, who will lightly keep her hand on you as she moves around the table. You are never alone in the dark, at the mercy of an unexpected touch or sound; your vulnerability is acknowledged, anticipated, managed, and calmed.

The same can be the norm with your patients and guests. Never let them feel they are alone, lost, vulnerable, without the immediate support of a caregiver, a valet or concierge, or transporter.

Keep a light touch on your patient when they are on a gurney or wheelchair, especially when they are out of the safety and comfort of their street clothes. Use a soft voice to reassure.

Instead of giving or pointing directions, accompany patients and guests to their destination. Then make certain they are personally acknowledged, received and handed off to another.

The CURSE of small numbers.

In small organizations, many processes and procedures will be performed so rarely that they will be hard to do efficiently, consistently, or well, and good outcomes and data will be hard to come by. Some of these procedures, especially those that are high risk, simply need to be transferred to larger, better prepared organizations, those that get the chance to routinely develop better and stronger skills.

This is a chance to bring in clinical experts for periodic in-service training, or partner with a best-in-class organization and offer rotations for skill development and experience.

You can't do everything well. No one does or can. Put the ego aside and do what is best for the patient.

Clinical DOCUMENTATION is a staff-wide commitment.

A garbage-in, garbage-out opportunity to avoid here, one to address with all clinicians: stress the necessity, the rules, and the importance of rigorous clinical documentation.

Every clinician knows they are not *paid* to treat patients—they are paid to document the care they provide. But one cannot exist without the other.

Business tools, including new and updated technology, create unending opportunities to learn new processes and standards. Requiring compliance is not enough. Create staff training opportunities, with easy to access tools and skill training programs, and allow time throughout the workday, especially remotely, to improve their performance.

Recruit a clinical documentation champion, someone who can connect with peers and users, to drive the success of a critical process throughout the organization.

INTEGRATE your clinical and financial data.

Here's a chance to use your patient care data to grow an excellent business.

With good and accurate clinical documentation and financial data sources, you can identify ways to improve clinical outcomes and develop a strong and accountable healthcare business for your community and market.

You can discover potentially unnecessary or inappropriate ER admissions, for example, and the chance to create patient specific urgent care centers, say for pediatrics or eldercare. Or you can uncover financial goldmines, such as athletics rehab or efficient home care opportunities.

And always, as every small business owner knows, you can and must discover recoverable market losses, for example with outpatient service access, with improved quality outcomes.

Improve the care and improve your bottom line.

Support the MID-LEVEL clinician.

Advanced practice and nurse practitioners, physician assistants, certified nurse midwives, and others: mid-level professionals can improve your organization's productivity, its safety and quality, and most importantly, can provide excellent patient care and engagement.

Embrace the benefit of these professional caregivers to enhance your core competencies. With shortages in primary care clinicians, they will prove invaluable. Include them as key members of your clinical staff. They will improve your business and quality. Patient satisfaction will soar.

Revisit the by-laws if necessary.

Technology doesn't SAVE any steps in the short term.

In fact, technological changes might make your organization's life more complicated and chaotic overall in the short term.

Implementing new technology resources will add to the burden of your organization in the short term, with implementation, training, resistance, and other concerns. Recognize and admit this; don't dismiss it.

Anticipate setbacks, chaos, pushback, and learning curves.

It won't be pretty, but it will be worth it.

Rollouts will suck the OXYGEN right out of the room.

Technology implementations and new initiatives can be relationship killers, or they can create beautiful friendships. EMR or Med Rec, new initiatives or innovations, or rebuilding projects, will simply take over the organization.

Knowing this, it's critical to find the right champion, the person with enough seniority and a good all-around reputation, to keep everyone focused, to remove roadblocks, to drive the project from start to finish without being easily distracted. Find someone who can establish strong, open lines of communication with vendors and consultants and organizational leadership. Find someone who can demonstrate the effectiveness and value of the new thing early and often.

Embrace BEHAVIORAL health.

Whether in the emergency department or your outpatient primary care clinics, behavioral health resources can enhance patient care management, enable appropriate care and hospital admissions, and improve continuity of care.

Strong partnerships between behavioral health and other clinical services can make patient transitions to and from the ED smoother, safer, and less fragmented.

Inpatient services can partner with behavioral health to support patient safety initiatives such as proper restraint management, difficult conversations, and reducing and dealing with hospital-induced dementia.

Above all, an integrated mental health program is worth its weight in gold to your continuum of care processes and your community.

LESS care
does not equal worse care.

Best practices and evidence-based clinical care processes can feel like takeaways. They aren't.

Listen to your staff and patients about their concerns with clinical processes that focus on providing effective care. You can dispel any notion that less invasive or intense care is worse care by welcoming their questions and giving expert answers.

Listening to and trying to understand why they may feel cheated out of all the care they think they need and deserve will give you the opportunity to address specific clinical as well as emotional concerns.

You can reassure them that with both yours and their newly acquired knowledge, best practice equals the best, the good kind of care they really deserve.

Create an inclusive CONTINUUM of care.

The hospital-centric model of healthcare has changed rapidly to a broader continuum of care, from acute, inpatient-based models to a network of outpatient, inpatient, and home-centered care. It's creating many more opportunities and avenues to provide and receive appropriate, cost-effective and best practice care.

Orient your business development to create an exceptional, inclusive network, especially at the service line (your small business incubators). These are fabulous opportunities to position your organization to best respond to and meet your customer's critical needs and expectations. It also takes advantage of all the clinical resources at your disposal.

Recognize your physician and CLINICAL partners.

Some clinical partners will be your key referral base, others are simply politically connected and valuable to the community, while others are just stinkers and always will be.

Get the scoop on your clinical partners, consider the sources of the information, and use the intelligence smartly and strategically to enhance your organization. They may be perfect partners in your continuum of care.

Many will be retiring or moving on, opening up gaps or opportunities to meet healthcare needs or patient access. Some may provide lessons in quality or excellence that you can always learn from; others can provide a chance to help deliver better care.

Recognize your clinical partners to enhance your quality of care and organizational excellence. It's good medicine.

Never forget
the FUNDAMENTALS.

This is healthcare, an industry that is a highly intensive endeavor of both clinical and human skills.

Your human skills were developed early and have evolved over your lifetime; your clinical skills are relatively new and will continue to develop during your working life, changing to reflect experiences, maturity, and new knowledge, training, and information.

In clinical care, run, don't walk, to take advantage of every opportunity to add to and learn fundamental skills and techniques, both deeper and broader, to serve your patients and your career.

Make the resources available to your staff and colleagues, including the necessary time and education funds, and encourage everyone's growth.

We are what we repeatedly do. Excellence, then, is not an act, but a habit.
Aristotle

Build COLLABORATIVE relationships.

Your organization's effectiveness as a network of care involves building strong professional relationships, including medical staff, nursing and physician assistants, clinical techs, social work, behavioral health, and every other member of the healthcare team.

Regularly revisit hospital and system by-laws and credentialing requirements to accommodate changes in best practice and financial care delivery models, to enhance staff collaboration and care delivery opportunities.

Build strong partnerships and relationships with even your closest competitor to improve patient access and to deliver the most effective, appropriate care.

Physician: HEAL thyself.

There's an old lawyer joke: What do you call a thousand lawyers chained together at the bottom of the ocean?

A good start.

Replace Lawyer with Physician here and you'll get the same nervous guffaws.

Physicians are the 800# elephant in the healthcare room, the sacred cow. They are the gatekeepers to healthcare: they control the access to inpatient care, outpatient treatment and referrals, pharmaceuticals, ancillary procedures, and so on. That's the reality. Outside of wellness and preventive care, physicians are virtually in control of the western healthcare system. Welcome outsized egos, financial and political power, and eventually exaggerated behaviors of entitlement and not uncommon bullying.

Much is made of efforts to improve relationships between physicians and others involved in healthcare; entire hospital and health system departments, not to mention consultants, are hired to teach communication skills, settle antagonisms, resolve conflicts, and soothe egos. It's a good start.

The reality is, it's time to stop the enabling: Physician, Heal Thyself.

Be good at what you do. Don't expect to be good at everything else too. Learn to play well with others. Everyone wants the clinical care done well, too. Don't bully or throw your weight around.

You can't do it alone. Become partners, not obstacles. Be the leaders you want to be.

Build centers of EXCELLENCE to be substantial.

Make your Centers of Excellence more than a bought and paid for credential or marketing tool.

Build your Centers of Excellence for substance. Then prove it to your community with quality, safety, best practices and data. Prove it over and over again to sustain it.

Exceed everyone's expectations, including your own.

Establish solid relationships with clinical EDUCATORS and professional schools.

Healthcare organizations frequently partner with clinical schools and programs to gain access to new care providers, from techs to nurses and other medical clinicians. These programs are good resources for future staffing needs, and provide career development opportunities for current staff.

But remember, when their students are on your floors, the students are *you*. They represent you with your patients, guests, and staff. Make sure they have the training they need *before* they arrive.

Not all schools or training programs are created equal. Before you partner with them, hold their instructors to your high quality standards. Keep them accountable for preparing their students with impeccable basic levels of clinical skills before they ever work with your patients and staff. Evaluate their students regularly; openly and honestly provide them with feedback for improvement.

And vice versa. Their success is a good test of your organization's commitment to quality, too.

Technology is a TOOL, not a goal.

Healthcare has slowly awakened to the incredible resource technology can be for clinical care and process improvement. Clinical care, patient records, communication, billing, accounting, best practice algorithms, materials management, human resources—the technology and equipment are there to handle it all.

And new mandates, regulations, and clinical processes have opened up reasons and opportunities to implement tech solutions, and ever more options and vendors are available to purchase and deploy.

Technology is a critical resource when used wisely and effectively. But beware: technological resources risk becoming expensive toys and sinkholes with financial, human, and time costs. Adapt tech tools wisely.

> The first rule of any technology...is that automation applied to an efficient operation will magnify the efficiency. The second is that automation applied to any inefficient operation will magnify the inefficiency.
> Bill Gates

11
Community

Build
COMMUNITY relationships.

The continuum of care that is 21st-Century healthcare means strong, open and collaborative relationships. It's a windy path for the most experienced professional, patient or healthcare customer, and utter madness for everyone else.

Work in partnership with the resources in your community to help your current and prospective patients and guests find their way to the most appropriate and meaningful care.

Research and dig for your data and that of your partners to uncover business solutions that can help you create optimal networks of care for your market—from referral sources previously untapped to gaps in the network that need to be filled to enhance everyone's health.

Be the leader of community OUTREACH.

Community outreach is an ongoing responsibility and chance for your organization to build upon its strengths.

From the relationships and activities needed to create an ACO or Medical Home, to defining your continuum of care, this is a no-brainer.

If you don't have one already, build a group or department to tackle your community outreach activities; to get to know not only your neighbors, but your partners and competitors as well as, especially, the immediate neighborhood.

Learn to see the healthcare community as they do, to view the gaps, the strengths or redundancies. Think of community outreach as a chance to improve healthcare access and efficiencies.

Become a good neighbor.

The CONTINUUM of care is best practice.

Build a system of care that extends beyond the walls of your facility. Establish solid relationships, partners and teams to give your patients and providers a solid network, a continuum of care resources and partners to provide for their ongoing needs.

Whether it's resources for preventive care, to referrals for specialized or home care, a continuum of care will help reduce expensive, inappropriate hospital admissions. Primary care, wellness, and urgent care resources are most effective for preventive care, for life's little but non-life threatening illnesses and mishaps, to chronic care management.

Outpatient surgical facilities and skilled nursing offer cost-effective care without the inconvenience, infection exposure, or unnecessary expense of inpatient hospital resources.

And homecare and hospice are always invaluable sources of care, comfort and quality for families and loved ones when ongoing rehabilitation or end-of-life issues are central in their decisions.

Your continuum of care is for all of life's healthcare needs.

How can we HELP?

Healthcare organizations are given the chance to be the heart and soul of the community. Most of what you do in your community is laced with emotion, which makes it inevitable that the opportunity to hold this honor is yours for the taking.

Here's your chance to step up to that challenge; to reach out and provide outstanding resources, relationships and partnerships; to actually live your organization's mission and vision at each stage and event of your community's life.

Step up and become part of your community, it's heart and soul.

Be a good NEIGHBOR.

When your grounds crew is shoveling the snow from the hospital's sidewalks, entrances, and driveways, how about continuing on along the street and shovel the entire block? Ditto for clearing the street gutters, parking strips, and the empty lots surrounding your facilities. They're probably not using shovels. So, be a good neighbor. Plow forth.

Provide adequate parking for your visitors and staff. Recognize the parking and space needs of your residential and commercial neighbors, and not just your own. Work with the local parking enforcement to establish appropriate access and accommodation.

Set an expectation of your staff that they treat the neighborhood respectfully.

Be a good neighbor.

Don't become the NIMBY. You're big, powerful and busy, so you can be gracious.

Grow a GARDEN.

Yes!

What a wonderful way to create and to build an environment committed to nurturing, care, peace and tranquility, and growth.

A community garden is not just a feel good project for your patients and guests. It is an incredibly potent message and space for your staff and neighbors, for the community you live and work in.

It's a metaphor. It's also incredible and valuable dirt between the fingers and toes.

It's a resource for growth, engagement, even fresh herbs and produce.

The smallest space will do the trick.

Listen for your community's PERCEPTIONS.

Here's one: Does your cafeteria double as a community center for the neighbors? If it does, that's a good sign. It's become the *third place*. It gives you an idea that the opinion of your local market is probably on the favorable side.

The same holds true with your community's older and long time residents; those who may feel a sense of ownership of your place, especially if they have grown up together. Take the time to listen to their stories.

Listen in on the grapevine in your community, the rumors that abound from your neighborhood partners, the foundation board, in the line at the grocery store. Listen to the hospital volunteers, even the pharmacists at the local box store.

Great ways to get to know what people are saying about you, what their perceptions are, and necessary to find out if you're going in the right direction. Just remember to use what you hear.

Make sure your community knows you are HERE, in a big, good way.

Be the go-to healthcare organization in your community.

From preventive and routine care, including education and on-line tools, referrals and advice on complementary healthcare resources, to end-of-life planning and care: be the first place your community turns for advice, connections, partnerships, the quality interactions that make their personal or professional lives work.

Even if you don't have what they need, be the place they turn to because they trust you to help them find it. Then do just that.

Be trustworthy, professional, resourceful, and easy to get to.

Make sure everyone knows you and can find you quickly when they need help. And long before they need you through the ED.

Become the best place to WORK.

Unless you are the only healthcare company in town, your clinical staff has a choice of employers. So too, especially, your non-clinical staff.

Take the time to figure out why people want to be, or don't want to be, part of your organization, why they stay and especially, why they leave. Research shows over again that, all things being equal, it isn't the pay or benefits or workload that make someone's workplace meaningful. It usually boils down to the leaders and colleagues who create a working environment and a workplace that are meaningful.

Be the best place to work, regardless of you status in the healthcare hierarchy, too. Whether its the neurosurgeon or the grounds crew, it's all about providing excellence to your community.

COORDINATE limited and scarce services.

When your clinical partners include rural, isolated, or unique and one-off services, build consortia to add a virtual or shared program to supplement onsite visits. The tools are available to enable big, wide programs to connect with professional colleagues for consultation, and with patients for follow-up, education and support. All at a fraction of the time, cost and inconvenience of personal visits and build-outs.

Improve access to scarce services and resources with technological resources, to allow your clinicians to deliver the best patient care; collaborate to build up your referral base; build system and care processes to ultimately demonstrate your best in class service, care, and compassion.

12
Sustainability

It's the SUBSTANCE that really matters, not the process.

Adopting new processes and initiatives to solve old problems and to perfect operations are exciting and energizing and may, finally, put you on the map.

If there's a solid ground for the new process to rest on, terrific.

If the substance, the core, is bad, however, a new process is just superficial: it's the Emperor's new clothes.

New ways of doing something that is fundamentally broken won't provide any long-term fixes. Band-aids and caulking will only work short-term before you'll eventually have to replace everything and build again.

Identify and value the substance of what you do; don't rely on the magic of a new process to make it better.

Change takes TIME.

Look out if you find yourself changing improvement processes often, either because the changes you want aren't happening quickly enough, or the group falls into a slump, or they just complain.

All change suffers through plateaus (think: exercise and diet) and groups can get restless and bored.

Find a tool that matches your mission, brand, image, and find opportunities to celebrate little but significant improvements, and stick to it.

It takes time for change, to gear up and get sticky. And it has to get personal. That takes time.

The whole is always GREATER than the sum of its parts.

Silos: Those ever-present cliques, scapegoats of healthcare and most old-order organizations.

What the ED does at any given time isn't related to what imaging or behavioral health does, is it? Except when it is related—which is most of the time.

Sound familiar? Rivalry, crisis management, inattention, ignorance. Why not change this outlook to one of collaboration and integration, and get a smooth running, well-oiled system of care, improving appropriate patient access, data-sharing, excellent clinical care processes and outcomes.

An excellent whole is always going to be a greater organization than the sum of its isolated parts.

The POWER of relationships.

Cross-functional collaboration, whether it is within the organization, with your community resources, even amongst competitors, is a resourceful way to share critical and meaningful experiences, legitimate information or data, and to build strategic alliances and innovation. It's the best way to deliver excellent patient care and improve the health of your community.

The power of relationships will let you create a continuum of care for your patients, clinicians and customers that will magnify the resources at their disposal.

It's another example of the whole being greater than the sum of its parts. It sustains your mission.

PLAY well with others.

Whether it's in-house service lines working to coordinate care, or competition between providers within your community, your patients and guests want to know they can rely on a consistently high quality of care, with seamless relationships and handoffs, when they need it.

Beware the professional jealousy, hostility, the petty badmouthing in the ranks. Patients and guests hear and feel everything, both directly and indirectly. They pick up on strained relationships. They know when there is bullying, backbiting, and just plain old not getting along. It sabotages your organization's goals. It ultimately, and most importantly, sabotages patient care.

So, commit to establishing and keeping your staff's relationships professional, respectful and calm. Find opportunities to bring key players together for a common cause: their organization's success and excellence.

LEVERAGE your resources and knowledge.

Being a good partner in your community involves contributing to its health, its success, and the success of its members. By partnering with local and regional vendors and suppliers, you contribute to the long-term health of the community, guaranteeing a stronger customer base for everyone.

From local products and supplies, such as food and operational resources, to collaborative relationships with local institutions like neighboring schools, utilities, government organizations and non-profits, banks, commerce, and others, you can set a standard for community commitment, support and overall good health.

Give everyone a chance to be an EXPERT at something.

Create new generations of leaders in your organization by giving staff a chance to become an expert, an authority, on something they do well.

It might be expert status with a new clinical application, a review or connection to the latest research, or teambuilding innovations, lessons learned at a seminar or class, or presenting their hard-earned thesis.

Let them teach their newfound expertise and skills to their group, their team, their peers and other leaders. Whether it's connections through such activities as brown bag lunches, book groups and science pubs: the list of opportunities to connect and share expert status is endless.

Grow your staff, encourage them to share their intellectual and energetic wealth, and create excellence for everyone.

YES, and . . .

One of the great and fun techniques taught in improvisation classes is to respond to your partner with "Yes, and..."

It's the way to keep the action going, to create forward motion, dynamic movement toward a solution.

What happens when you say "no?" Everything stops. No movement, no action. The action just drops to the floor.

Try using "Yes, and..." in your work environment. It creates positive, forward motion and, not surprisingly, helps build stronger relationships and solutions, with coworkers, patients and guests of all kinds.

Try it out.

Move from data-fest to ACTION.

Know what to measure, when to measure, what it tells you, and when to pull the trigger on using what you know and how to use it.

Ask "So what?" at the beginning of every query. Data for data's sake? Even the best pure researchers know when to stop gathering data and get on with it.

If you can't answer the "So what," stop gathering data. You either have more than enough, or you have the wrong kind, you're asking the wrong questions.

Build GREEN. Work green.

Everyone is expecting it: Your staff, guests and patients, peers, neighbors, partners, even regulators.

LEED, sustainable building and operational practices, eco-friendly products and processes, alternative energy and resources, food service and environmental care, the list goes on and the resources to adapt sustainable practices are growing daily.

Building and operating green is not a fad; it's the new normal.

The first law of ecology is that everything is related to everything else.
Barry Commoner

Take exceptional care of your FRONTLINE.

Customer service, random and illogical changes, care-giving, bullying, competing tasks, and the inability to leave the scene to regroup can all add to the stress, anxiety, and burnout of the frontline staff.

Value your frontline for their best work, their time, intelligence and insight.

Build space and opportunities into their day to escape and decompress, to make sure they are able to continue to provide the attention and best patient and guest care everyone deserves.

Allow your frontline to thrive in their work, to feel respect and appreciation, and to guarantee they can sustain the compassion needed to care for your guests and patients from their first contact.

Create spaces to ESCAPE.

Healthcare screams checklists, reports, endless documentation—all-important and critical to sustaining quality patient care.

What it doesn't give much attention to is the downtime and quietude that is necessary for critical thinking, time-consuming thought work. To relieve anxiety and stress. To deal with grief.

How wonderful to create spaces for staff, clinicians, patients and guests, to check out during breaks or periods of stress.

Whether it's in a community garden, the solarium, or a quiet chapel, make room and space for your people to decompress, refresh and reinforce themselves.

Fit all of the PUZZLE pieces together.

What do the emergency department, the lab, patient admitting and environmental services have to do with each other? Everything that's important: Patients visiting the ED frequently end up as inpatients, by way of lab results, by way of the admitting physician, by way of the patient registrar, and by way of the availability of clean rooms.

When these pieces of the organization don't fit together like a puzzle, the patient will get stuck in the ED for time immemorial and everyone gets mean, mad, grumpy, and patient care and safety suffer.

When these services work together well, the patient is in the bed on the floor and in the care of the appropriate clinician in the quickest, most efficient way possible.

Everyone is happy, cared for, and getting healthy.

Get it? It's a good feeling when the pieces fit.

SUCCESS.

Success is growth and sustainable margins, of course.

Success is confident leaders and staff; transparent planning; excellent outcomes and accomplishments.

Success is a calm and well-tended environment.

Success is solid and respectful relationships, collaborations, and communications amongst the clinical and non-clinical staff.

Success is patient and guest trust and cooperation.

Care what your people THINK.

We all want to be heard. We all are the Stars in our own play.

Your employees are hired for their competence and skills, for their potential to make things great. They want to feel empowered to do what they do best, and they want to be recognized for it.

Your employees are your front line—they see what is going on, what the patient sees and wants, and they know what works, what doesn't.

Listen to your people, trust them, and care what they think. They know what's going on.

Technology TRAINING, from A to Z.

Technology changes rapidly. Some of your staff will be more proficient and eager to learn than others, in spite of their job requirements.

Don't assume your staff knows everything they need to know about the technology and tools you ask them to use. Ask if they know how to use the applications you require, but don't do it in a group setting. No one likes to admit in front of their peers that they don't know how to download an attachment from their smartphone, not to mention reattaching it after they've done with it what was required.

No one likes to look stupid; we get plenty of chances to do that on our own time. Provide space and attention to work it out in private.

To ensure up to date capability and compliance, especially with new products and rollouts, offer basic to advanced tech training opportunities to everyone, throughout their tenure with your organization. Set up tutorial workstations in lounges, libraries, even remotely. Recruit super-users. Keep everyone up to speed.

Build career and SUCCESSION planning into your strategic plan.

Do members of your staff need to move out of the organization in order to move up and grow their careers? Do you primarily hire cheap, young college grads, those eager to take on the world, but who are likely to leave in a few years for graduate school, relieving you of the need for career development resources? Thought so.

How much good talent are you losing that way? Many jobs and professions in healthcare are limited by virtue of specialized training, but there are opportunities for the best to continue to contribute. Don't lose your stars, your core players. Prepare them and your organization for the future.

Do it all AGAIN tomorrow.

And the next day.

And the day after that.

Acknowledgments

Thanks to Hann and Sam for your love, support, and patience.

Thanks to the red peanut M&M on the floor in the sterile hospital hallway, the one that kept me moving, even when it hurt, and kept me coming back to visit. Wonder where it went?

And thanks to every one of you who read this and make excellent and innovative things happen in the healthcare world.

Go to it!

About the Author

A P Palmer has worked in the healthcare industry for over 15 years, alongside some of the highest quality, as well as some of the not so great, physicians, hospital executives, politicians and consultants in the country. With graduate work and experiences in public health, international development, and starting from a roundabout tour through architectural design, she has developed a keen eye for innovation and improvement, and fitting the puzzle pieces together.

Notes, ideas, words, and brainstorms:

www.ingramcontent.com/pod-product-compliance
Lightning Source LLC
Chambersburg PA
CBHW031836170526
45157CB00001B/324